Learning to Learn
in Nursing Practice

Kath Sharples

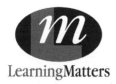

LearningMatters

First published in 2009 by Learning Matters Ltd

British Library Cataloguing in Publication Data
A CIP record for this book is available from the British Library

ISBN: 978 1 84445 244 6

Cover design by Toucan Design
Project Management by Diana Chambers
Typeset by Kelly Gray
Printed and bound in Great Britain by TJ International Ltd, Padstow, Cornwall

Learning Matters Ltd
33 Southernhay East
Exeter EX1 1NX
Tel: 01392 215560
E-mail: info@learningmatters.co.uk
www.learningmatters.co.uk

FSC
Mixed Sources
Product group from well-managed forests and other controlled sources
Cert no. SGS-COC-2482
www.fsc.org
© 1996 Forest Stewardship Council

before

Learning to Learn
in Nursing Practice

Series Editor: Shirley Bach

Transforming Nursing Practice – titles in the series

To order, contact our distributor: BEBC Distribution, Albion Close, Parkstone, Poole, BH12 3LL. Telephone 0845 230 9000, email: **learningmatters@bebc.co.uk**. You can also find more information on each of these titles and our other learning resources at **www.learningmatters.co.uk**

Contents

Foreword

If you are a student on a nursing course, or improving your learning in practice skills, the process is exciting and challenging in equal measures. It's exciting because there are new things to learn which will bring riches as an academic award or career opportunities. It's challenging because you are expected to follow a course that has hardly a moment to spare. One minute you are in the classroom and the next you are in a ward full of very ill or recovering patients, or perhaps spending time with a person who needs gentle patience and understanding to support them through a distressing experience. The juxtaposition of experiences and variation is an essential part of the learning landscape. Kath Sharples offers you, in this book, the tools to manage your learning as you travel across that landscape.

An overview of the historical background to the pre-registration course will help you understand why your learning is guided by the NMC standards and the importance of learning in practice. The book explores the differences between your approach to learning as an adult to that as a child, and the impact your previous learning experiences can have on your learning now. Sections on the vital role that mentors play, how you can work with them to support your learning, and the importance of assessing your own learning style to get the best from practice learning will help you make the most of your time.

Preparing for your practical learning is an investment. The book demonstrates how you can plan for your personal needs and different situations. A key to making your learning work for you will be your drive, determination and motivation. Practice environments will provide you with a wealth of different learning experiences. Your own enthusiasm for taking each of those experiences and turning them into a learning opportunity will be your strongest ally. In this book you will find many strategies, underpinned with practical examples and research, to assist you complete the competencies you will need in your course. There may be challenges ahead; however, the tactics you need to 'learn to learn' are here and will help you achieve your ambition.

Shirley Bach
Series Editor

Acknowledgements

Thanks to Mel, Lyn and Anne, my colleagues in the Practice Education Support Unit, Thames Valley University, who provide endless support always.

Thanks to Karen Elcock (Practice Education Support Unit, Thames Valley University) whose passion for practice education is a constant inspiration.

Thanks to the pre-registration nursing students at Thames Valley University who teach me something new every day.

Thanks to Di Page for her encouragement and Becky Taylor at Learning Matters for her constant words of wisdom, and for making the whole process enjoyable from beginning to end.

Special thanks to Ann for her belief, encouragement, support and love.

Kath Sharples

The author and publisher would like to thank the following for permission to reproduce copyright material:

Dennison, B and Kirk, R, *Do, Review, Learn, Apply: A simple guide to experiential learning*. Copyright © 1990, Blackwell Education, Oxford. Adapted Figure 2.7, 'The Johari window', p29, reproduced with kind permission of Blackwell Education.

Honey, P and Mumford, A, *The Manual of Learning Opportunities*. Copyright © 1989, Peter Honey Publications, Maidenhead, UK. Adapted table on 'Conscious Learning', p1, reproduced with kind permission of Peter Honey Publications, Maidenhead, UK.

Honey, P and Mumford, A, *The Manual of Learning Styles*. Copyright © 1992, Peter Honey Publications, Maidenhead, UK. Adapted learning cycle diagram, p. 7 and Learning Styles text extract, pp5–6, reproduced with kind permission of Peter Honey Publications. The publisher would like to note that *The Manual of Learning Styles* is now out of print and has been replaced by Honey, P and Mumford, A, 2006, *The Learning Styles Questionnaire, 80-item version*, Peter Honey Publications, Maidenhead, UK.

Kolb, David A, *Experiential Learning: Experience as the source of learning and development.* Copyright © 1984, p42. Figure 3.1 adapted by permission of Pearson Education Inc., Upper Saddle River, NJ.

Pattison, D, Parsons, D and Weatherhead, C, Connecting reflective practice with clinical supervision, in Ghaye, T and Lilliman, S (eds) *Effective Clinical Supervision: The role of reflection*. Copyright © 2000, Quay Books, Salisbury, Wiltshire.
Adapted text extract, p76, reproduced with kind permission of Quay Books, MA Healthcare Ltd.

Introduction: Your training – your career

Congratulations on choosing a career in nursing. You are training to enter a very special profession that very few other professions can equal. By reading this book it can be assumed that you wish to improve your ability to learn in, through and during practice placements. Perhaps you are at the beginning of your training programme and wish to prepare for that first experience of being 'in practice'. Or maybe you have progressed in your training and are looking for ways to hone your ability to learn 'in practice'. Whatever the reason, rest assured that this book is for you. Not only is there advice for practice learning, it will also help to allay common fears, and perhaps even correct some misconceptions related to the clinical environment you may have. Essentially, this book will be a guide for what to learn in practice, how to learn in practice and when to learn in practice.

The standards to be a nurse

The standards that you need to reach in order to qualify as a registered nurse have been set for you by the Nursing and Midwifery Council (NMC). The *Standards of Proficiency for Pre-registration Nursing Education* (NMC, 2004) contains a list of specific competencies that you must achieve in order to progress in your course. The first progression point is from the Common Foundation Programme into the Branch Programme. The second progression point is for entry into the professional register. In order to achieve a competent standard at each progression point, you will need to demonstrate that you have the skills to learn in practice.

The *Essential Skills Clusters for Pre-registration Nursing Programmes* (NMC, 2007) also contains a list of specific competencies that you must achieve in order to progress in your course. Once again, the first progression point is from the Common Foundation Programme into the Branch Programme. The second progression point is for entry into the professional register. In both cases, there are competencies that are dependent on, and link to, your ability to learn in practice. The following boxes contain these specific competencies.

STANDARDS OF PROFICIENCY FOR ENTRY TO THE REGISTER: PERSONAL AND PROFESSIONAL DEVELOPMENT

1. Demonstrate a commitment to the need for continuing professional development and personal supervision activities in order to enhance knowledge, skills, values and attitudes needed for safe and effective nursing practice.

Outcomes to be achieved for entry to the branch programme

Demonstrate responsibility for one's own learning through the development of a portfolio of practice and recognise when further learning is required

- identify specific learning needs and objectives
- begin to engage with, and interpret, the evidence base which underpins nursing practice

Acknowledge the importance of seeking supervision to develop safe and effective nursing practice

Standards of proficiency for entry to the register: personal and professional development

- identify one's own professional development needs by engaging in activities such as reflection in, and on, practice and lifelong learning
- develop a personal development plan which takes into account personal, professional and organisational needs
- share experiences with colleagues and patients and clients in order to identify the additional knowledge and skills needed to manage unfamiliar or professionally challenging situations
- take action to meet any identified knowledge and skills deficit likely to affect the delivery of care within the current sphere of practice.

2. Enhance the professional development and safe practice of others through peer support, leadership, supervision and teaching.

Standards of proficiency for entry to the register: personal and professional development

- Contribute to creating a climate conducive to learning.
- Contribute to the learning experiences and development of others by facilitating the mutual sharing of knowledge and experience.
- Demonstrate effective leadership in the establishment and maintenance of safe nursing practice.

(NMC, 2004, p34)

ESSENTIAL SKILLS CLUSTERS – CARE, COMPASSION AND COMMUNICATION

---

1. Provide care based on the highest standards, knowledge and competence.

Outcomes to be achieved for entry to branch

- Uses professional support structures to learn from experience and makes appropriate adjustments.

Outcomes to be achieved for entry to the register

- Uses professional support structures to develop self-awareness, challenge own prejudices and enable professional relationships, so that care is delivered without compromise.

(NMC, 2007, p2)

2. Provide care that is delivered in a warm, sensitive and compassionate way.

Outcomes to be achieved for entry to the register

- Through reflection and evaluation demonstrates commitment to personal and professional development.

(ibid., p6)

Lifelong learning

In order to meet these standards at each stage of your course, you will need to develop the accompanying skills that make learning in practice possible. Most notably, in order to qualify as a nurse, you will need to demonstrate the ability to learn as an adult. In fact, the NMC requires that all nursing students in the UK develop lifelong learning skills throughout their training, and are competent lifelong learners at the point of qualification.

> *The rapidly changing nature of healthcare reflects a need for career-wide continuing professional development and the capacity not only to adapt to change but to identify the need for change and to initiate change. The provision of safe and effective healthcare and appropriate responsiveness to the changing needs of services and patients or clients cannot be achieved by adhering to rigid professional boundaries. The standards of proficiency must, therefore, include the capacity to extend the scope of practice and to address lifelong learning skills within all programmes of preparation.*
>
> (NMC, 2004, p14)

This means that the NMC will only accept that you are a competent nurse if you are also a competent learner. Not only will you need to demonstrate that you are able to learn during your training, but you will also need to demonstrate that you have the skills to continue learning for the rest of your professional career.

Book structure

In Chapter 1, 'Practice learning in the pre-registration nursing curriculum', we begin the learning journey by looking at a brief history of your pre-registration nursing curriculum. We will explore how and why decisions were made regarding the purpose and nature of practice learning, and the relevant NMC standards that impact upon your practice learning experience.

In Chapter 2, 'Learning as an adult', we take a look at adult learning theory, and its relevance to your practice learning experiences. You will have the opportunity to identify the key aspects of adult learning theory and gain an understanding of the main characteristics of adult learning. We will also consider the implications of your prior learning experience and how this may impact on your ability to learn as an adult.

In Chapter 3, 'Your mentor in practice', we will explore the role and responsibility of your mentor in terms of your practice learning experience and the assessment of your competence. We will identify the accountability and responsibility of a mentor in relation to the NMC standards for mentorship and the mentor's role in facilitating your learning. We will also look at the factors that mentors must consider when undertaking your assessment in practice and determining your competence, including the role of the sign-off mentor in relation to your practice support.

In Chapter 4, 'Learning with style', we take a look at your learning style and the way that you learn. There will be an opportunity to understand how your own learning style fits within your personality, and also to match your learning style with the types of clinical activities that suit your style of learning. We will also delve into the importance of engaging with all learning styles in order to develop competence in practice.

In Chapter 5, 'Preparing for clinical placement', we will clarify the specific preparation you will need to undertake prior to the commencement of your practice placement. Not only will you have an opportunity to identify the key aspects of practice preparation, but you will also be challenged to consider the relevance of specific placement preparation in terms of your personal needs and the practicalities involved in planning confidently for your learning experiences.

In Chapter 6, 'Self-regulated learning in practice', we will develop a clear understanding of the theory behind, and purpose of, self-regulated learning in practice. There will be a chance to explore the main principles of self-regulated learning and the specific challenges of learning in practice. The relationship between self-regulated learning skills and the role of your mentor will be investigated as a means of achieving competence.

In Chapter 7, 'Learning through experience', we will take a practical approach to the use of self-regulation to learn in, through and during your clinical experiences. We will discuss the link between self-regulated learning and learning through experience. We will investigate how to use a learning cycle in order to plan your placement learning experiences, and how reflection can be used to learn from placement experiences.

In Chapter 8, 'Learning through feedback', we will discuss the role of feedback in relation to your learning experience and assessment of competence. The chapter will be focused on identifying the key aspects of verbal and written feedback, understanding the relevance of the feedback in facilitating learning, and the role of the mentor in delivering feedback.

In Chapter 9, 'Learning to learn in practice', we will identify the role that motivation plays in your practice learning experience, and the potential obstacles to learning that you may encounter. We will discuss various factors that affect motivation, the difference between intrinsic and extrinsic motivation, and common threats to motivation within clinical practice. We will also explore a number of strategies you can use for getting and staying motivated to learn in practice.

Learning features

The skills you will need to develop for learning in, through and during your practice experiences are explained throughout this book. There will be practical advice throughout, including preparing for your practice learning experience, and learning through personal experience and feedback. You will have the opportunity to develop your own learning skills by engaging with a number of practical exercises and reflecting on your own experiences. There is also a glossary at the back to assist you with unfamiliar terms. Glossary terms are in bold in the first instance that they appear.

This book cannot do the learning for you; however, by understanding more about practice and your role in practice you will develop confidence for learning to learn in nursing practice.

1. Practice learning in the pre-registration nursing curriculum

CHAPTER AIMS

The aim of this chapter is to explore the recent developments of the pre-registration nursing curriculum and how this will impact on your practice learning experience.

After reading this chapter you will be able to:

- identify the key development stages of the current pre-registration nursing standards and proficiencies;

- understand the relevance of NMC standards in relation to pre-registration nursing and your practice learning experience;

- make sense of your pre-registration nursing programme in relation to the structure and content of your practice placements.

Introduction: starting to learn

Most student nurses begin their nurse training with lots of questions about their training and very few firm answers. Many of these questions are regarding the practice learning element of the programme. If this sounds like you, then rest assured you are not alone. Taking any university course can be daunting; however, the nursing course can add a whole new dimension to your stress as the requirement to spend 50 per cent of your training 'in practice' can take you right out of your comfort zone.

ACTIVITY 1.1

Have a look at the list of questions below. Do you know the answers? Have you ever considered these questions before?

- Who decides what I need to learn to be a nurse?
- Who decides on the content of my programme?
- Who makes the decisions about my learning in practice – where I go, what I do and how long I do it for?
- What will be expected of me in practice?

The questions in Activity 1.1 may have occurred to you before, or this may have been the first time you have questioned anything about your nursing course.

Whatever the case, it doesn't really matter. What does matter is that you find out the answers to all these questions. This is because your whole nursing programme and, specifically, the practice element of your training is based on the answers to these questions. The aim of this chapter is to begin to answer these initial questions that you may have regarding your practice learning. We will start with a quick history lesson in relation to nurse education, and then we will move on to the role of the NMC in relation to your nursing course. There will be an opportunity to identify the key requirements of your practice learning experience and how your nursing programme will have been designed to meet these requirements. There will also be an opportunity for you to investigate your overall nursing programme structure and clarify when clinical experiences are likely to occur.

A quick history lesson

In the 1980s, nurse education in the United Kingdom (UK) transferred from hospitals to universities. This decision was made after years of consultation undertaken by the United Kingdom Central Council (UKCC). The grand plan for the future of nurse education in the UK was outlined in a document called *Project 2000: A new preparation for practice* (UKCC, 1986). This was a very dramatic change and caused quite a lot of controversy. Many people were against moving nurse education into universities; however, the decision was made following much criticism of the then methods of preparing future nurses (UKCC, 1999). The reality was that many other countries in the world, such as the USA and Australia, had already moved to university training for nurses. So it was really only a matter of time until the UK did the same. Many people felt that UK nurses would be left behind if they did not adopt the same training approach as the rest of the world. The goal was to prepare nurses for a career of changing roles, lifelong learning and continuing professional development (CPD) (UKCC, 1999). As a result, the apprenticeship style of nurse training was abandoned in favour of university-based education.

Project 2000 involved many important decisions and issues being discussed by the UKCC regarding how nurses were to be trained. One of the issues involved the amount of time that students would spend in theory learning and practice learning. Another issue was related to the role of student nurses during their practice experience. The move into university training meant that student nurses were no longer to be regarded as part of the workforce. However, when the original *Project 2000* curriculum was implemented during the early 1990s, the final 20 per cent of a student's time in practice was known as **rostered service** (UKCC, 1986). As a result, students were counted in workforce numbers.

The implementation of rostered service caused some notable problems. While this approach may have been advantageous in terms of staffing levels, it did not provide student nurses with the best possible learning experiences. Many students found that, instead of being given additional learning opportunities and responsibility, they were more likely to be delegated the role of nursing assistants. As a result, students were finishing their nurse training unprepared for the accountability and responsibility of a registered nurse. In light of this development, one of the key recommendations within the *Fitness for Practice* report (UKCC, 1999) required that students be provided with consistent clinical supervision in a supportive learning environment during all practice placements (ibid.). This effectively extended the **supernumerary** status for students to include the whole of the programme.

RESEARCH SUMMARY

Fitness for practice

In 1998, the UKCC undertook an urgent review of the standards for pre-registration nursing and midwifery programmes in the UK. Chaired by Sir Leonard Peach, the Commission for Education was given the following remit:

> *To prepare a way forward for pre-registration nursing and midwifery education that enables fitness for practice based on healthcare need.*
>
> (UKCC, 1999, p6).

The report highlighted that there were numerous problems associated with pre-registration nursing programmes, and that there was disturbing anecdotal and empirical evidence that newly qualified nurses and midwives required constant support, raising questions regarding fitness for practice at the point of registration. The report highlighted that problems associated with the organisation and supervision of practice placements, in conjunction with work pressures and the pace of healthcare environments, were hindering the development of practice skills.

As a result, the *Fitness for Practice* report included a number of recommendations for changes to the delivery and structure of practice placements within pre-registration nursing programmes. Most notable among a host of recommendations were the following:

> *Recommendation 10*
> - *That the standards required for registration as a nurse be constructed in terms of outcomes for theory and practice.*
> - *That the standards required for registration as a nurse specify that consistent clinical supervision in a supportive learning environment during all practice placements is necessary.*
>
> (ibid., p37)

In addition, the report highlighted that assessment of a student's competence during practice placements could not be reduced solely to an assessment of a student's ability to carry out certain tasks. In other words, there was a requirement for students to demonstrate their competence through work, rather than an emphasis on performance during task-based work. The report saw the birth of a new term; **'knowledgeable doer'** became synonymous with the concept that pre-registration nursing programmes should not only prepare students for fitness for practice at the point of registration, but also should provide them with the higher-order intellectual skills and abilities for life-long learning (UKCC, 1999).

Being supernumerary

The term 'supernumerary' is one of the most controversial and misunderstood terms within nurse education in the UK. Originally, the term was intended to mean that students would be viewed as additional to the numbers of staff already employed in a clinical area. Students were given supernumerary status in order to ensure that they were free to learn, and engage with the best and most appropriate learning opportunities for their level of training. It was never intended that students would no longer involve themselves in work while on practice placement. Unfortunately, over time, the meaning of the word has became confused, and students and nurses alike have interpreted 'supernumerary' as implying that students are to observe practice rather than participate in work during practice placements.

The reason for this confusion is unclear; however, this is possibly due to some nurses and students falsely assuming that, as students were no longer to be considered part of the workforce, they would not be participating in 'work'. This misconception still exists in many practice areas today, and some students also continue to perpetuate the myth that they are on practice to observe only. This is quite clearly incorrect, and students who believe this do themselves and their colleagues a disservice. So, once and for all, let's get it clear. According to the NMC:

> Supernumerary status means that the student shall not as part of their programme of preparation be employed by any person or any body under a contract of service to provide nursing care.

> (NMC, 2004, p19)

Put quite simply, this means that, as a student, you are to be considered additional to the numbers required to deliver safe nursing care within a clinical area. This means that you will have the freedom to learn *through* work on practice placements. It does not mean that you are to take on an observation role only, as quite clearly it is just not possible to learn in this way.

The significance of the decision to grant students supernumerary status cannot be overestimated. This one decision has had an enormous impact on the learning opportunities and experiences available to you today. The way you learn in practice now, and your opportunities for learning, all stem from the fact that you are supernumerary and, in essence, have been awarded the freedom to learn. The NMC has recently reinforced the supernumerary status of students by clarifying that, while you are on practice placement, you are not required to be under a contract of service to provide nursing care (NMC, 2004). In Chapter 9 we will look at supernumerary status in far more detail, including the ways in which you can use supernumerary status to maximise your learning opportunities. However, for the time being we need to take a closer look at who is currently in control of your nursing programme.

The NMC

On 1 April 2002, the Nursing and Midwifery Council (NMC) replaced the UKCC as the regulatory body for nurses and midwives in the UK (NMC, 2004). As a result, it is now the NMC that decides on the core content of the pre-registration nursing curriculum and the overall structure of the programme. Obviously, the main recommendations from the *Fitness for Practice* report (UKCC, 1999) have been revised over the years, although many of the key principles still feature within current programme guidelines. In keeping with this, from time to time the NMC will review their current standards and recommendations for nursing education in the UK. Changes are usually made after consultation exercises that can last many years and are based on feedback from a wide range of sources, including nurses and students. At the moment there are two main documents that contain the standards for pre-registration nursing education in the UK. These are the *Standards of Proficiency for Pre-registration Nursing Education* (NMC, 2004) and the *Essential Skills Clusters for Pre-registration Nursing Programmes* (NMC, 2007). The relevance of these two documents to your overall training programme has already been outlined within the Introduction to this book. However, it is worth having a quick review of the major features of these two documents in light of your practice placement experiences.

Standards of Proficiency

The *Standards of Proficiency for Pre-registration Nursing Education* (NMC, 2004) have been provided by the NMC to guide your university on the structure and nature of your nursing programme. It is the current gold standard for how nurses are to be trained in the UK, and sets the criteria that all universities must follow. By providing these standards, the NMC is able to control and monitor the quality of the nursing programme you receive. It also ensures that, no matter what university you attend, you will be receiving a pre-registration training programme that is of equal quality to all nursing students in the UK. These proficiencies are not negotiable and your university will have had to provide evidence to the NMC of how your training programme supports the standards they have set.

Within the *Standards of Proficiency*, the NMC lists 12 separate standards related to your programme, with additional guidance on how universities should meet these standards.

STANDARDS OF PROFICIENCY FOR PRE-REGISTRATION NURSING EDUCATION

The NMC has provided your university with a comprehensive list of guidelines that it must follow in order to provide your nursing programme. The key areas for which the NMC provides instruction include:

- the length of your nursing programme;
- the structure of your nursing programme;
- the balance of theory and practice within your course;
- the teaching and learning strategies that should be used in your course;
- the academic standard of your nursing programme;
- the content of your course;
- the support you should be offered while on the course;
- the nature of the experiences you should receive during the programme;
- how your branch programme should train you for your intended area of practice;
- the types of knowledge that should be explored to underpin practice;
- the types of assessment strategies that should be used during your course;
- your supernumerary status.

As you can see, the areas covered by the *Standards* are very comprehensive and many of them relate specifically to your experience of learning in practice. The following are just some examples of the types of instruction that the NMC provides to your university in relation to your nursing programme.

Instructions from the NMC

- The balance of learning must be 50 per cent practice and 50 per cent theory in both the Common Foundation and Branch Programmes.
- Your practice experience should include opportunities to experience 24-hour/7 days a week care of patients.
- No practice placement should be less than four weeks in duration.
- Students should be supported in practice learning environments.
- Students must be assessed in practice against the *Standards of Proficiency* for entry to the register.
- Practice experiences should be educationally led and supernumerary status maintained.

It is also important to understand that the NMC does not just make recommendations that will fulfil requirements for your registration as a nurse.

The guiding principles of the *Standards of Proficiency* are aimed at ensuring that you are prepared for the future requirement to be a lifelong learner. As a result, the document outlines the standards that are expected of students at two specific points in their nursing programme. Throughout your nursing course these standards will be used to make a judgement regarding your competency. The first stage or competency level lists the standards you must achieve in order to move from your Common Foundation Programme (CFP) into your Branch Programme. The second stage indicates the standards you must achieve by the end of your Branch Programme in order to enter the professional register at the completion of your training. Not only must you be prepared in order to meet 'fitness for practice', but your course should also prepare you in terms of **fitness for purpose**. It will be expected that, at the point of qualifying, you are able to relate to the changing needs of the health services where you work in terms of current and future needs. A core principle of this agenda is the focus on students being prepared for ongoing professional development. In the words of the NMC: *The* Standards of Proficiency *must include the capacity to extend the scope of practice and to address lifelong learning skills within all programmes of preparation* (NMC, 2004, p14).

Essential Skills Clusters

As we discovered when looking at the *Standards of Proficiency* (NMC, 2004), there is a little room for flexibility in the structure of your programme as long as the underlying principles are met. This is why different universities have different ways of teaching the nursing course; while the delivery and content of your course may differ slightly from that of students at other universities, the end goals are basically the same. The same cannot be said of the *Essential Skills Clusters for Pre-registration Nursing Programmes* (NMC, 2007).

The *Essential Skills Clusters* are determined by the NMC and also lay down very clearly the standards that are expected of students at the two specific points of their nursing programme: competence for entry to the Branch Programme and competence for registration. For each stage there is an explicit criterion that must be fulfilled, with each criterion listed within a specific 'cluster'. In total, there are five clusters, as follows.

ESSENTIAL SKILLS CLUSTERS DOMAINS

1. Care, Compassion and Communication
2. Organisational Aspects of Care
3. Infection Prevention and Control
4. Nutrition and Fluid Management
5. Medicines Management

Source: NMC (2007).

Throughout your nursing course you will be assessed according to these standards in both the theory element of your course and the practice element. It is therefore highly recommended that you take the time to read the entire *Standards of Proficiency* and *Essential Skills Clusters* documents if you have not already done so. They are quite lengthy; however, they also clearly outline the level of proficiency you must meet at the end of your CFP and also to qualify as a nurse. You will be able to put the various elements of your training and individual course requirements into context by taking the time to absorb these documents.

Learning in clinical practice

It should come as no surprise that the NMC also sets the standards for the support and assessment you receive during your practice placement. The *Standards to Support Learning and Assessment in Practice* (NMC, 2008) make these expectations very clear, and the majority of your learning experiences in practice will be guided by these standards. We will take a much closer look at these standards and the role of the mentor in Chapter 3. For the time being though, it is worth noting that these standards exist and that, ultimately, the NMC governs every aspect of your practice learning.

Curriculum design

Curriculum design is a really important aspect of your nursing programme. The course you are doing (or perhaps thinking of doing) was written and designed by lecturers from your university, and the process will have taken many months. The whole curriculum will be based on an agreed philosophy of learning and teaching, so that all elements of the programme can be traced back to the same core values. In addition, the curriculum will have been designed to ensure that the requirements outlined by the NMC in the aforementioned *Standards of Proficiency* (NMC, 2004) and *Essential Skills Clusters* (NMC, 2007) can be met.

SCENARIO

Imagine that you have just bought a wonderful plot of land and decide to build a brand new house. You start by finding out the building regulations and agreeing the architect's plans. The building work starts with the foundations and then moves on to the general structure. Once these are in place, you add in key features such as walls and floors so that each main section is clearly defined and follows a logical sequence. You gradually add in more and more detail using your own creative style, for example buying furniture for specific rooms and choosing paint colours. When the house is finished it is inspected to ensure that it meets building regulations and complies with the required standards. Once this has been done it is ready for occupation and you can enjoy it and all its benefits.

Building a nursing curriculum

In some ways, designing a nursing curriculum is a little bit like building a house. The building regulations are like the NMC standards, and the blueprints for the curriculum can be creative but must comply with the underpinning regulations. The foundations will be based on a philosophy of adult learning, so that all the internal structures of the curriculum are based on that structure. Quite obviously, it is not until you have an understanding of how the whole curriculum will look that you can start to focus on the specific areas. If you tried to build a house by concentrating on the small details first, you would quickly run into trouble, for example furniture that didn't fit the rooms. It is the same principle that underpins a nursing curriculum.

Validation

Once your university had designed the nursing curriculum, they would have asked the NMC for final approval of the course. The NMC would have sent a team of inspectors out to your university to pore over the curriculum plans. They would have looked at all the documentation to ensure that it met their standards and guidelines. When satisfied with the curriculum, the NMC would have validated it. This would have been the final seal of approval that was needed before the curriculum could be taught.

My curriculum

Now that you have an understanding of how your pre-registration course was designed and the elements it must contain, it is important to look at the overall structure of your nursing course. In particular, it is worthwhile for you to understand the structure of your practice placements, where these will be spent and how long you will spend in each one.

ACTIVITY 1.2

Below, you will find a grid that you can use to document the structure of your pre-registration curriculum. There is an opportunity to outline both the theory and practice elements. Each year is clearly defined so that you can easily identify the individual elements and how these may alter as you progress through the course. Try to include as much detail as possible, for example the module titles, how long each module will be and at what stage in the year it will occur. If you can, include the number of hours you will be required to complete for each module.

Year 1 – Common Foundation Programme

Module title	Theory element	Practice element

Year 2 – Branch Programme

Module title	Theory element	Practice element

Year 3 – Branch Programme

Module title	Theory element	Practice element

It is not uncommon to find that some modules will contain no practice element, and some modules will contain no theory. However, no matter what the structure or design of your curriculum, you can be assured that it will comply with NMC standards and contain the required elements to expose you to the full range of learning experiences set by the NMC.

CHAPTER SUMMARY

In this chapter we looked at the recent history of nursing education in the UK, and the current implications of this for practice learning. The range of standards set by the NMC in relation to the pre-registration curriculum was outlined, along with a brief overview of curriculum design and validation processes. We discussed that, in order to make the most of learning opportunities available to you during clinical practice, you will need to understand the structure and content of the theoretical and practical aspects of your curriculum.

KNOWLEDGE REVIEW

Having completed the chapter, how would you now rate your knowledge of the following topics?

	Good	Adequate	Poor
1. The key development stages of the current pre-registration nursing standards and proficiencies.			
2. The relevance of NMC standards in relation to pre-registration nursing and your practice learning experience.			
3. Your pre-registration nursing programme in relation to the structure and content of your practice placements.			

Where you're not confident in your knowledge of a topic, what will you do next?

Further reading

Nursing and Midwifery Council (NMC) (2004) *Standards of Proficiency for Pre-registration Nursing Education.* London: NMC.
Available from **www.nmc-uk.org**. Outlines the specific requirements of your nursing course as instructed by the NMC, including the standards of competency you must achieve throughout your training.

Nursing and Midwifery Council (NMC) (2007) *Essential Skills Clusters for Pre-registration Nursing Programmes.* London: NMC.
Available from **www.nmc-uk.org**. Outlines the standards of competency you must achieve throughout your training.

Useful website

www.nmc-uk.org All standards documents listed within this chapter can be easily accessed and downloaded on the NMC website.

2. Learning as an adult

CHAPTER AIMS

The aim of this chapter is to explore the relevance of adult learning theory in relation to expectations of your learning in practice.

After reading this chapter you will be able to:

- identify the key aspects of adult learning theory;
- understand the main characteristics of adult learning;
- consider the implications of prior learning experience for your adult learning ability;
- identify your main expectations and assumptions as an adult learner in practice.

Introduction: adult learners

From the minute you enrolled on your nursing course there were certain expectations of you, and assumptions made about you related to your learning. Your tutors will expect that you have the ability to be an adult learner and they will have developed your course on the assumption that you will be able to learn as an adult. The implication is that if you are not prepared to learn as an adult, then you may struggle with various learning situations, especially the practice element of your course. It is very important, therefore, to understand the expectations and assumptions of you as an adult learner so that you are able to gain the best possible learning experience during your practice placements.

This chapter will first consider what an adult learner is, before looking at the main theories and assumptions about how adults learn – assumptions that your course is likely to be based on. Then it will explore some of the factors that may impact on your ability to learn as an adult, before finally looking at how this relates to what will be expected of you in practice.

Can I learn?

In our current culture it is generally accepted that anyone, irrespective of age, has the capacity to learn (Dawson, 2006). While you may agree with this statement, it is worth considering that this belief has not always been held in the past. It was not so long ago that the concept of adult learning was met with some scepticism. There have been numerous myths and misconceptions regarding the impact of ageing and the capacity to learn (Hayes, 2006), and statements such as

'You can't teach an old dog new tricks' have probably perpetuated such myths. However, Withnall et al. (2004) conclude that, while the ability to learn may diminish or be erratic with age, a fit and healthy person continues to learn new things throughout adulthood.

It is important to keep in mind, however, that how you learned as a child does change when you become an adult learner. Adults see the world very differently from the way a child does, and this will affect everything that you do, including the way you learn. The techniques and strategies that you used when you were very young will not automatically work for you as an adult. When you were a child some of your education would have been focused on teaching you the skills to make learning possible. From an early age you have been exposed to learning how to learn. It is now time to continue this process by learning how to learn as an adult.

Characteristics of an adult learner

Let us start by looking at some of the characteristics of adult learners.

- *They are above the age of compulsory education.*
- *They have some experience of the world of work.*
- *They have family responsibilities.*
- *They have financial responsibilities.*
- *They have domestic responsibilities.*
- *They are reasonably independent.*
- *They are able to make their own judgements about the world around them.*

(Corder, 2008, pp4–5)

Does this list describe you and how you function in the world? If so, then you are officially regarded as an adult learner. You can easily see from the list that being an adult learner does not just relate to your age, but also concerns your relationships, responsibilities and how you relate to the world. The fact that you are an adult learner, however, does not automatically mean that you will have no problems learning as an adult. Just as it was when you were a child, you will need to learn *how* to learn as an adult.

How do adults learn?

So we now know that having the characteristics of an adult learner does not automatically result in the ability to learn as an adult. Over the years there have been many theories about the ways in which adults learn, and the elements within an educational programme that produce the best environment for learning. The specifics of such theories are beyond the scope of this book and will not be dealt with in any great detail. If you want to know more about adult learning theories, there are some suggestions for further reading at the end of this chapter. It is important, however, for you to understand the general principles of adult learning that have guided the development of your nursing curriculum.

The andragogical learner

Your nursing programme will have been designed to meet the needs of the adult or **andragogical** learner. Think back to our housebuilding scenario in Chapter 1 (see page 13). Adult learning theory (andragogy) is just like the blueprint or plans for building the curriculum. Everything about your curriculum, therefore, is designed to build a nursing course for you as an adult learner. There is nothing new about this approach, as Malcolm Knowles' theory of andragogical adult learning began to gain momentum around the 1970s and continues to be a popular approach in adult learning today.

Andragogy is a term that describes an organised and sustained effort to assist adults to learn in a way that enhances their capacity to function as self-directed learners (Mezirow, 1983). In other words, it is a way of teaching adults that suits the ways in which adults naturally like to learn. At its core the andragogical approach to adult learning recognises that adults have a unique set of motivations for learning (Rogers, 1983). For example, children have very little choice regarding their learning, as education is a legal requirement between certain ages. Adults who are involved in learning, however, are doing so by choice rather than force. No one has made you do your nursing course; you choose to do this for reasons that are important to you. For this reason, the main feature of the andragogical approach is that it encourages adults to use their skills of **self-direction** and their life experiences in order to learn (Howard, 1993). It recognises that adults do not always enjoy being told what to do, and like to use their previous knowledge and experience to work things out for themselves. This means that, as an adult learner, you will be given the opportunity to learn independently in certain areas without the need for constant formalised tuition (Timmins, 2008). As your practice learning experiences will be based on principles of adult learning theory, you should expect that independent learning will feature within your clinical placements.

SCENARIO

Karl has arranged a trip to a museum. There is an exhibition of Picasso paintings that he has been wanting to see for years. He has been looking forward to this so much that he bought a book on Picasso three weeks ago so that he could understand the background to the paintings selected for the exhibition. He also looked up the museum website and booked tickets to the curator's talk on the paintings. When he arrives he collects an audio guide and takes his time wandering through the exhibition. The book has given him valuable insights into the paintings and the audio guide adds so much more to his experience. The curator's talk is excellent, and he is able to understand so much more of what is said because of his prior knowledge. Karl has enjoyed the whole day and can't wait to share his experiences with his friends.

Can you see that Karl has approached his whole day as an adult learner? He decided to see the exhibition because he was genuinely interested in it. However, he also took responsibility for ensuring that the experience was enjoyable. He did some prior research and arranged to attend a talk. He could have just turned up, as there was no one telling him what to do, but he would have been the one to miss out. By taking the initiative, Karl was able to enjoy and learn far more from the experience.

Assumptions about the adult learner

There has been much debate regarding adult learning theory over the years, but there are five core principles that have remained consistent and are viewed as the gold standard of understanding how adults learn. These in turn have led to some assumptions regarding adult learners. Let us start by looking at these five core principles.

Core principles of adult learning

- *The adult learner wants to be self-directed.*
- *The adult learner accumulates over time a reservoir of experience.*
- *The adult learner has a readiness to learn.*
- *The adult learner is aware of their own learning needs.*
- *The adult learner is motivated to learn.*

(Knowles, 1984, 1989, 1990; Knowles et al., 1998)

It is very important that you understand the significance of these core principles and assumptions about adult learners. Did you know that these assumptions will have been made about you? Your nursing course will have been designed based on the assumption that you are an adult learner and that you embrace at least some of the core principles of adult learning. If any of these core principles are lacking, then you may well struggle to learn in the context of an adult learning course.

ACTIVITY 2.1

It is worth taking the time now to reflect on your abilities as an adult learner. Each of the core principles we looked at earlier has been rephrased into a statement about you. Try reading each statement out loud and consider whether this is an accurate description of you.

- I want to be self-directed.
- I have over time accumulated a reservoir of experience.

- I have a readiness to learn.
- I am aware of my own learning needs.
- I am motivated to learn.

How did you get on in Activity 2.1? Were there any statements that you cannot relate to? In order for each statement to be true, you will need to think of evidence to support each of these statements. For example, how have you demonstrated your readiness to learn? If you are aware of your learning needs, what are they? You see, at the same time as your university may be assuming that you have the qualities required of an adult learner, you may also have assumed that you have these qualities. However, you can't just assume that they exist – there needs to be proof. If you cannot think of examples within each of these criteria, this may be because, at the present time, they do not exist. If this is the case, don't worry – each of these qualities can be learned.

Positive and negative experiences

While there is no doubt that you are an adult, it may be that you are not yet totally prepared to learn as an adult. There can be numerous reasons for this. It is not uncommon for people to have had negative experiences related to learning. Rogers (2007) suggests that, for some people, their experience of school education has been disappointing and perhaps even associated with ritual humiliation. If this has been your experience, these memories can be quite powerful and can affect your ability to learn as an adult. Dawson (2006) refers to this as the 'baggage' of our previous learning experience.

Not all of your experiences will have been negative, however. There will have been times in your life when you were successful in learning new skills or gaining knowledge. Unfortunately, the memories of negative learning experiences may overshadow your accomplishments. You may feel that you have to repair the damage done from the past before you can learn again (Corder, 2008). In fact, you may be reading this book because you believe that you lack the ability to learn in practice. If your past experiences of learning have been negative, it may be your self-belief that needs an overhaul, rather than your ability to learn.

CASE STUDY 2.1

Naimh is a mature-age nursing student on her first clinical placement. It has been over 20 years since she last did any formalised study, although she has participated in a number of short courses at an adult learning college in recent years. Naimh begins the placement full of enthusiasm, but she is very nervous as she wants to make a good impression.

In her second week she is attending to the personal care of a client with a learning disability. He is very agitated and begins to hit his head against the bathroom wall. She calls for help and her mentor comes to her aid. The mentor knows the client very well and uses a variety of communication techniques to calm him down. Later on that day, Naimh's mentor asks her if she has been taught any communication techniques during her nursing course. While the remark was not meant to be critical, Naimh feels devastated. She is taken straight back to her school years, when she was accused of being slow and regularly humiliated by teachers. She assumes that her mentor now thinks she is stupid and she leaves the room crying, her confidence shattered. Her mentor cannot understand what she has done wrong; she had only wanted to discuss with Naimh some communication strategies and had decided to begin by asking Naimh what she had been taught so far on her course.

Naimh has brought into her brand new learning situation painful memories of her past that have not been resolved. The mentor has no knowledge of this, so a simple conversation is interpreted by Naimh as criticism. In order to move on, Naimh will need to make the transition from an adult learning as a child to an adult learning as an adult.

Putting learning into perspective

If your self-belief about your ability to learn has taken a battering over the years, you will need to repair this before you begin your practice learning. If you doubt yourself and lack confidence, you will not be able to make the most of your learning experiences. Let us start by getting one thing straight: no matter what your educational background or prior experiences, you are capable of enjoying the buzz of learning something new (Corder, 2008). The fact is that we learn all the time, throughout our entire lives. Some learning is formalised, for example at a college or university, and this type of learning may lead to a qualification. Quite a lot of learning that you do, however, may be quite informal, and you may not even recognise it immediately as learning. It is very easy to trivialise this type of learning, assuming that it doesn't matter, or is not as important or as impressive as the formal types of learning. All learning is important, however, and every time you learn something new you prove to yourself that all learning is possible for you.

ACTIVITY 2.2

Have a think about the range of skills that you already have, that you learned as an adult. Now use the box below to note down all of these skills. Be honest about your accomplishments and don't put yourself down. For example, you may be able to surf the internet or fly a kite. Perhaps you can repair a bicycle puncture or create a song list on your iPod. It doesn't matter how trivial you may think your achievement is, the fact is you have learned something, so be proud and write it down.

```
┌──────────────────────────────────────────────────────────────┐
│                                                                │
│   Skills that I have learned:                                  │
│                                                                │
│                                                                │
│                                                                │
│                                                                │
│                                                                │
│                                                                │
│                                                                │
└──────────────────────────────────────────────────────────────┘
```

Take a very good look at all the things you have written in Activity 2.2. You had to learn all these skills. Over the course of your life you have continued to develop and learn new skills, and every time you add another thing to the list you prove to yourself that you can learn and, more importantly, can learn as an adult.

Adult learning in practice

It is time to face up to the fact that there will be certain expectations of you when you begin your practice placement. First, it will be expected that you will possess at least some ability to learn as an adult. You can, therefore, expect to be treated as an adult learner. For example, it will be assumed that you will have some ability to be self-directed and self-motivated in your learning experiences. As a result, your opportunities to engage with the best possible learning experiences will depend on your ability to be self-directed and self-motivated. Do not worry if you are unsure about what this means or how to go about doing it, as there are chapters in this book that will deal with all these issues. At this stage, all you really need to do is understand why these expectations exist.

Second, you can expect to have mutual responsibility for planning your own learning, rather than it being planned for you. Unlike learning that you may have experienced as a child, you will not be given specific instructions for every learning experience. It will be assumed that you will be able to seek out and plan some of your learning experiences independently. This may come as quite a culture shock, especially if this is your first exposure to an adult educational programme (Knowles et al., 2005).

The focus of this book, therefore, will be on how to develop the skills of an adult learner in practice. Remember that, in order to qualify as a nurse, you will need to demonstrate that you are competent in practice, and practice learning will be the proof of your competence. It may be worth looking once again at the *Standards of Proficiency for Pre-registration Nursing Education* (NMC, 2004) and the *Essential Skills Clusters for Pre-registration Nursing Programmes*

(NMC, 2007), as these make expectations for your competence very clear. We will, therefore, be focusing on how to learn, how to plan for learning, and how to gain the most from each learning opportunity. Along the way you will gain insight and hopefully the skills of self-motivation, self-regulation and reflection on your learning. You will be learning to learn in nursing practice.

CHAPTER SUMMARY

While everyone has the ability to be an adult learner, it is also true that not all adults will be prepared to learn as adults. It may be that there is a need to overcome negative learning experiences from the past in order to develop the skills of an adult learner. Throughout your nursing course it will be expected that you are able to learn as an adult. You must come to terms with the assumptions and expectations of you as an adult learner in order to develop your ability to learn in, through and during practice. This may require you to develop your motivation and self-direction in practice.

KNOWLEDGE REVIEW

Having completed the chapter, how would you now rate your knowledge of the following topics?

	Good	Adequate	Poor
1. The key aspects of adult learning theory.			
2. The main characteristics of adult learning.			
3. The implications of prior learning experience for your adult learning ability.			
4. Your main expectations and assumptions as an adult learner in practice.			

Where you're not confident in your knowledge of a topic, what will you do next?

Further reading

Dawson, C (2006) *The Mature Student's Study Guide*. Oxford: How To Books.
This book offers some great advice and tips for studying as an adult.

Knowles, M, Holton, E and Swanson, R (1998) *The Adult Learner*, 5th edition. Houston, TX: Gulf.
A useful text for explaining in detail the principles and application of adult learning theory.

Useful website

www.mind.org.uk/Information/Booklets/How+to/How+to+increase+your+self-esteem.htm This is an easy, user-friendly website that explains the fundamentals of poor self-esteem and reasons why self-esteem may fluctuate and, most importantly, gives some practical advice for improving your self-esteem.

3. Your mentor in practice

CHAPTER AIMS

The aim of this chapter is to clarify for you the role and responsibility of your mentor in terms of your practice learning experience and assessment of your competence.

After reading this chapter you will be able to:

- identify the accountability and responsibility of a mentor in relation to the NMC standards for mentorship;

- understand the mentor's role in facilitating your learning;

- explain the factors that mentors must consider when undertaking your assessment in practice and determining your competence;

- recognise the requirements of the sign-off mentor role in relation to your practice support.

Introduction: learning in practice

In the previous chapter we dealt with the primary expectations of you as an adult learner. However, it is also likely that you will have some expectations related to the type of support *you* should receive while on practice placement. Obviously, learning is a two-way process and, in many ways, your learning will be related to and directly affected by the quality of the learning environment in which you undertake your practice experience.

The aim of this chapter is to help you understand the nature of the practice environment, the role of your **mentor** and the factors related to practice support. We will start by considering your current understanding of how your role in practice fits with the mentor's role. Next, we will examine the standards the NMC expects of mentors and also the type and nature of support your university is required to provide for you in practice. The role of the mentor will then be looked at in some detail, as well as your mentor's accountability. The additional support mentors can access is then covered, and the chapter ends by looking at the new role of sign-off mentors.

Expectations of practice learning

Before you can even begin to learn in practice, you will need to have a very clear understanding of what your role is in practice and how this fits with your mentor's role. The student grapevine is notorious for turning myths into what seem like facts, so for this reason it is very likely that you may have heard stories or information about practice learning that are untrue and therefore incorrect. If this is the case, your expectations of your mentor in relation to practice learning will also be incorrect. False assumptions tend to lead to false conclusions. The problem is that, if you attend practice placement with incorrect expectations and false assumptions, the consequence can be an unfulfilling and negative experience. The starting point, therefore, is to begin by looking at the real facts regarding practice placement, and hopefully dispel once and for all some common myths along the way.

ACTIVITY 3.1

No doubt you will have some beliefs about your practice placement and what you can expect from your mentor. Use the space below to finish the sentence about the expectations you have in relation to your mentor. List as many things that you feel your mentor should provide for you during your placement.

I expect that when I am on clinical placement my mentor will . . .

_____

_____

_____

_____

_____

For the time being you don't have to do anything with this list. However, from time to time during this chapter you will be asked to come back and refer to your list to remind yourself of your expectations.

NMC standards regarding practice support

The list you have made in Activity 3.1 will contain the support you expect to receive from your mentor. What you may not realise is that the NMC has already decided on the level of support mentors are required to provide for you. The NMC has set very clear guidelines regarding this support, and these guidelines are listed in the *Standards to Support Learning and Assessment in Practice* (NMC, 2008). These standards were first published in August 2006 and came into force on 1 September 2007. In July 2008 the standards were updated, and right now these are the current guidelines that your mentor is expected to follow. Importantly for you, one section of these NMC standards states that you must be provided with appropriate support from your university and also the practice area while you are on placement. Thus, while you may have your own personal expectations, it is actually the NMC that sets the criteria and expectations for your support and assessment during your practice placement.

University support

In Chapter 1, on page 11, we identified that practice learning equates to
50 per cent of your total training. In reality, this means that 2,300 hours of your
training experience will be spent in practice. The NMC makes it very clear to
your university that students should be supported in both academic and practice
learning environments (NMC, 2004). In order to ensure that you are adequately
supported in practice, your university is required to audit the practice learning
environment to identify the number and nature of students that may be
effectively supported (ibid.). This is to ensure that the practice area where you
complete your placement is the right sort of environment for your learning
needs. These reviews are carried out yearly and your university is required to
submit these reviews to the NMC when quality inspections are undertaken.
There are many factors that are taken into consideration when deciding on
whether a clinical area can and should support students during their clinical
placements, and your university and the clinical area will make these decisions
in partnership.

The role of a mentor

While you are on clinical placement, your day-to-day support during the practice
experience is undertaken by a mentor. Therefore, it is very important that we
now take the time to look at the specifics of a mentor's role and responsibility in
far more detail, paying particular attention, in this section, to how your mentor
should fulfil their role.

Who is a mentor?

Let us start by defining who a **mentor** is, based on the NMC definition:

*An NMC mentor is a registrant who, following successful completion of an
NMC approved mentor preparation programme, has achieved the knowledge,
skills and competence required to meet the defined outcomes.*

(NMC, 2008, p19)

This means that, first and foremost, your mentor must be a registered nurse, and
must have completed and passed an NMC-approved mentorship course in order
to gain a mentorship qualification. From this point on, a mentor is professionally
bound to adhere to the *Standards to Support Learning and Assessment in
Practice* (NMC, 2008).

Mentor support

Once qualified, the NMC requires mentors to support learning in practice in a
variety of different ways. These can be found in the above-mentioned standards
(ibid.) and have been summarised as follows.

- To provide support and guidance to students when learning new skills or
applying new knowledge.

- To act as a resource to the student to facilitate learning and professional growth.
- To directly manage a student's learning in practice to ensure public protection.
- To directly observe a student's practice, or use indirect observation where appropriate, in order to ensure that NMC-defined outcomes and competencies are met.

Therefore, as the name would suggest, your mentor's role according to the NMC standards is to support your learning and to support your assessment. We will look at each of these aspects in turn.

Support of learning in practice

The NMC makes it very clear that your mentor is required to co-ordinate appropriate learning experiences for you during your placement. This is quite a substantial role and involves both of you working together in partnership to ensure that you are provided with realistic and appropriate experiences. Both you and your mentor will need to have a very good understanding of your learning goals in order to choose and maximise the best range of learning experiences.

ACTIVITY 3.2

Take the opportunity now to look back at the list you created in Activity 3.1 regarding the expectations of your mentor.

- Are your expectations focused on the facilitation of your learning?
- Have you written anything that suggests that your mentor will be supportive of your learning?
- If so, are your expectations accurate and realistic, based on what you now know about the Standards to Support Learning and Assessment in Practice (NMC, 2008)?

It is likely that you may have listed an expectation that your mentor will act as a teacher during your placement. If so, then take note that this is inaccurate and unrealistic. It is the type of myth that is assumed by students to be fact. However, the NMC makes it very clear that your mentor is not required to be your teacher. Some students find this a very difficult concept to grasp, and have an expectation that their mentor will allocate time to undertake 'teaching'. On the contrary, it is expected that, as an adult learner, you will be more inclined to engage with facilitation of learning experiences rather than relying on didactic teaching. We will have the opportunity to explore this further in

Chapters 6 and 7, where we will discuss self-regulated learning and experiential learning. In the meantime, it is worth having a look at the accountability and responsibility of mentors within the *Standards to Support Learning and Assessment in Practice* (NMC, 2008).

ACCOUNTABILITY AND RESPONSIBILITY OF MENTORS

- *Organising and co-ordinating student learning activities in practice.*
- *Supervising students in learning situations and providing them with constructive feedback on their achievements.*
- *Setting and monitoring achievement of realistic learning objectives.*
- *Assessing total performance – including knowledge, skills, attitudes and behaviours.*
- *Providing evidence . . . of student achievement or lack of achievement.*
- *Liaising with others . . . to provide feedback, identify any concerns . . . and agree action as appropriate.*

(NMC, 2008)

Facilitation of learning

It is very clear from this list that the NMC requires your mentor to be focused on the facilitation of your learning, rather than teaching. In fact, 'teaching' per se is not mentioned at all. This concept fits in very neatly with the notion of an adult learner that we dealt with in Chapter 2. Remember that, as an adult learner, it will be expected that you will take mutual responsibility for your learning, rather than expect it to be done for you. You will have an opportunity to discover ways in which you and your mentor will be engaging with learning experiences described in Chapter 7.

CASE STUDY 3.1

A mentor speaks about their experience of facilitating student learning:

I actually love being able to mentor a student on placement. It's really rewarding when you have a student who is just so keen to learn everything they can, and you're able to see them becoming more confident as they develop their skills with the patients. It keeps me on my toes as well, especially when we discuss a patient's care plan or treatment. The last student I had asked me something about a new procedure I'd never heard of and that was great; we ended up learning something new together.

The main point is that you should attend practice placement with a very clear understanding of what it is you would like to learn and the types of experiences you would like to engage with in order to fulfil your learning outcomes. The NMC then requires your mentor to co-ordinate and facilitate appropriate learning opportunities according to your individual needs.

Learning takes place through the feedback you receive. This means that the real driver of your learning is you. If you attend a practice placement without a clear understanding of your learning objectives, your mentor will have nothing to facilitate. The risk is that, with no clear objectives, you may be seen as an extra pair of hands rather than as a learner (Johnson and Preston, 2001).

CASE STUDY 3.2

Elizabeth is a third-year student and is on clinical placement in a children's day-care unit. By the second week of placement, several mentors have noticed that Elizabeth seems to lack motivation and, on a number of occasions, she has been late back from her lunch break. She has been offered opportunities to assess children coming into the unit and develop her own treatment plans, but she seems reluctant to work independently and sits down regularly at the desk. When Elizabeth attends the daily planning meeting she does not ask to be allocated her own patients, and prefers to shadow her mentor throughout the shift. Elizabeth's mentor decides to question her regarding her motivation as she is clearly unhappy. Elizabeth explains that she is unhappy because she is not learning anything on the placement.

Her mentor cannot understand this comment and reminds Elizabeth that she has been offered responsibility every day for her own patients: to admit them into the unit, plan, manage and deliver care, and organise discharges throughout the day. 'Oh I know,' says Elizabeth, 'but I'm not learning – no one is teaching me anything.'

Support of assessment in practice

The second role that your mentor must fulfil during your clinical practice is to assess your competence. When you arrive at the clinical placement you will already have been provided with a set of learning objectives. It is your mentor's job to assess you on these objectives during your clinical placement. The learning opportunities that you engage with during your placement will provide your mentor with an opportunity to observe your practice and make a judgement about your competence. Your mentor is required by the NMC to assess your total performance in order to determine competence (NMC, 2008).

Have a look at Figure 3.1 on p32. This represents the three aspects of competence that you will be assessed on for each of your learning outcomes. You will note that all aspects of competence are of equal importance, so your knowledge, for example, is no less or more important than your professionalism or skill. It is

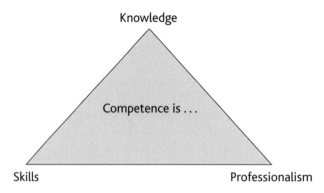

Figure 3.1: What is competence?

very important that you understand that your competence will be judged not just on what you can do (skills; also known as psychomotor skills), but also on what you know (knowledge; also known as cognitive skills) and the way you act (professionalism; also known as affective skills). Just as we discussed in Chapter 1, you must prove to your mentor that you are a 'knowledgeable doer'.

How competent do I need to be?

The competence level that you will be expected to meet has been set by the NMC and outlined within the *Essential Skills Clusters for Pre-registration Nursing Programmes* (NMC, 2007) and the *Standards of Proficiency for Pre-Registration Nursing Programmes* (NMC, 2004). We first looked at the contents of these documents when examining the design of your pre-registration curriculum in Chapter 1 and also in the Introduction to this book, so it may be worth referring back to these to refresh your memory. The fact is that all your learning outcomes will be related to the competency level expected of you at each stage of your nursing programme. It should come as no surprise, therefore, that both of these documents also contain information related to your practice assessment and the role of your mentor. In fact, no matter what stage of the programme you are on, your mentor will be required to assess you against NMC standards, whether this is to progress on your course or to qualify as a nurse.

Mentor accountability and responsibility

Your mentor is also accountable and responsible to the NMC for all the assessment decisions they make about you. The following statement in the *Standards to Support Learning and Assessment in Practice* (NMC, 2008) makes this very clear:

> *Mentors will have been prepared to assess student performance in practice and will be accountable for their decisions to pass, refer or fail a student.*
>
> (NMC, 2008, p32)

The NMC provides each university with very clear guidelines on the structure and nature of your practice assessment. In turn, your university will provide you with a practice assessment document that is based on these guidelines. Your mentor is professionally obligated to follow this assessment process, as the NMC will hold them accountable for the assessment decision they make about you. The assessment process that your mentor is required to follow means that they must provide evidence of your achievement or lack of achievement during your clinical placement.

Feedback on competence

Typically, the evidence of your competence that your mentor must provide will be in the form of documented notes within your practice assessment document or portfolio, and verbal feedback throughout your placement. This is to ensure that you are kept well informed of your progress. However, the feedback is not just for your benefit. At the end of your placement the NMC requires your mentor to document your progress within an 'Ongoing Achievement Record'. This is to allow comments and feedback from your mentor to be passed on to your next placement in order to enable your next mentor to make judgements on your progress (NMC, 2008).

The feedback you receive, both written and verbal, is an essential aspect of your learning experience, so we will deal with this subject in far more depth in Chapter 8. For the time being, it is important to understand that the provision of feedback is not optional, and the NMC requires your mentor to do this because it is fundamental to your learning. The documentation that your mentor provides within your assessment document also furnishes evidence that your assessment has been undertaken fairly, accurately and according to assessment guidelines. Without such documentation there is no proof that your assessment has met the required standards set by the NMC.

Additional practice support

If your mentor has concerns about your progress on a practice placement, the NMC requires them to seek help. Some students find this particular aspect of the mentor role very difficult to understand and this can lead to them feeling that they have been betrayed by their mentor. However, it is very important to understand that your mentor is not your friend, but your assessor. This is not to say that your mentor should not be friendly; but their role is functional and does not have the same features, functions or attributes as a friendship.

From the time your placement begins, your mentor is under significant pressure to make an accurate and objective assessment decision regarding your competence. They just cannot afford to get this wrong. If they require help in their mentoring role, the NMC makes it very clear that they should ask for it.

Georgiana has just passed her driving test and decides to buy her first car. She spends a whole weekend looking through magazines, searching the internet and walking around car dealerships. By the end of the weekend she has some idea about the best car to buy, but decides to get some help from others before making her final decision. Her best friend, Dorothy, has driven a similar model before and is able to share her experiences. Her grandfather, Keith, is a retired mechanic and offers to go with Georgiana on another test drive. Her brother, Michael, has had recent experience buying his own car and gives her some advice regarding finance options. After making use of all this advice and support Georgiana is far more confident about her decision and becomes the proud owner of her first car.

The point of the above scenario is that, when important decisions need to be made, it is good practice to share your dilemma with someone else who can offer a different perspective and may be able to suggest alternatives that have not yet occurred to you. The value of someone else's opinion when faced with a difficult problem is often invaluable. The same can be said for mentors who are concerned about your progress.

Support for mentors

The support your mentor may access can include other mentors, practice teachers, practice facilitators or link tutors from your university. They may ask for assistance with the facilitation of your learning experiences, action planning or assessment strategies (NMC, 2008). Your mentor can also ask that other members of the teaching and healthcare team contribute to your learning and assessment in practice; however, they alone will be accountable and responsible for undertaking the summative assessment of your learning outcomes (NMC, 2004). It is reasonable, therefore, to expect that a range of people may be involved with the facilitation of your learning, discussing your progress and assessment of your competence.

ACTIVITY 3.3

Now look back once again at the expectations you had of a mentor at the beginning of this chapter.

- Think about the expectations you had of your mentor in relation to assessment, learning and feedback.
- How have your expectations changed?

Based on what you have learned in this chapter, you may find it useful to use the space below to write your new expectations.

I expect that, when I am on clinical placement, my mentor will . . .

_____

_____

_____

_____

_____

Sign-off mentors

By now you should have a very clear understanding of your mentor's role in relation to your practice learning. However, in order to safeguard the health and well-being of the public, the NMC must be assured that, at the end of their programme, pre-registration nursing students have been assessed and signed off as capable of safe and effective practice (NMC, 2008). As a result, the NMC has decided that the mentor who makes the final decision regarding your competence for registration must fulfil additional criteria, and will be called a **sign-off mentor**.

How will the sign-off mentor role affect you?

It is very important to understand if and when the sign-off mentor role will affect you. If you began your nurse training after 1 September 2007, you will need to be assessed on your final placement by a sign-off mentor. The exact placement for which you will require a sign-off mentor will depend on the length of your course of study and the programme you are on, so you will be kept informed of this by your university. Needless to say, practice areas throughout the UK are currently developing their mentors to be sign-off mentors in order to ensure that there are adequate mentors for all final placement nursing students.

When you are being assessed on your final placement by a sign-off mentor, it is important to understand that the criteria for your assessment will not change, and neither will the criteria you will need to demonstrate in order to achieve competence. It will mean, however, that your mentor should be given protected time to provide feedback when undertaking their mentoring role, as this will be made possible under the mandatory time specification for sign-off mentors (Sharples, 2007b). Keep in mind, though, that, as the fundamental aspects of mentorship, facilitation of learning and assessment of competence remain unchanged, the sign-off mentor role will be an adjunct, rather than a change, to your practice experience.

CHAPTER SUMMARY

The role of the mentor is very clearly defined within the *Standards to Support Learning and Assessment in Practice* (NMC, 2008). In order to make the most of your learning opportunities while on practice placement, it is very important that you have clear and accurate expectations of your mentor. In this chapter we have looked at the role of the mentor in relation to both your learning experience and assessment of competence. The criterion for assessment of competence has been addressed, as has the professional obligation of a mentor in terms of written and verbal feedback. Additional support for mentors during a student's practice placement can promote objective assessment and, as such, is an NMC requirement to support learning and assessment.

KNOWLEDGE REVIEW

Having completed the chapter, how would you now rate your knowledge of the following topics?

	Good	Adequate	Poor
1. The accountability and responsibility of a mentor in relation to the NMC standards for mentorship.			
2. The mentor's role in facilitating your learning.			
3. The factors that mentors must consider when undertaking your assessment in practice and determining your competence.			
4. The requirements of the sign-off mentor role in relation to your practice support.			

Where you're not confident in your knowledge of a topic, what will you do next?

Further reading

Nursing and Midwifery Council (NMC) (2008) *Standards to Support Learning and Assessment in Practice: NMC standards for mentors, practice teachers and teachers.* London: NMC.
The NMC standard is quite a long document, but it does provide a comprehensive overview of the professional accountability and responsibility of mentors.

Useful website

www.rcn.org.uk/search?queries_search_query=MENTOR+TOOLKIT The RCN
mentor toolkit can be downloaded from the RCN website. The toolkit offers tips and
advice for mentors on facilitating your learning experiences while on placement.

4. Learning with style

CHAPTER AIMS

The aim of this chapter is for you to gain insight into your learning style and the way that you learn.

After reading this chapter you will be able to:

- understand how your own learning style fits within your personality;

- match your learning style with a range of clinical activities that suit your style of learning;

- understand the importance of engaging with all learning styles to develop competence.

Introduction: my style of learning

In Chapter 2, 'Learning as an adult', we established that everyone has the ability to learn. We also discussed that some students doubt their ability, possibly as a result of previous experiences that may have undermined confidence. If this has been your experience, hopefully by now you will have had the chance to dispel some old myths and boost your self-belief in your ability to learn. However, the ability to be a successful learner takes more than self-confidence. Before you can even begin to start learning, you will need to understand how you, as an individual, learn. This chapter will first look at how adults learn and what we mean by learning styles. It will then look at how this relates to your own learning style, and what your learning style might be. Next, there will be an opportunity to discover the approaches to learning that suit you best, based on your learning style, and how this might be used during your practice placement. Finally, the chapter looks at what to do if a learning situation does not match your personal preference.

Learning styles

The first thing to understand about the way you learn is that it is unique to you. This is generally referred to as your 'learning style' and is linked to various aspects of learning, such as the way you concentrate, process, internalise and remember new information (Dunn and Dunn, 1999). In fact, because the way you learn is a part of your personality, it would be very unusual for your learning style to exactly match someone else's. This also means that the way you learn, the way that works best for you, has developed over many years, although you probably were not aware that it was happening.

Lifelong learning

Throughout your life you have been learning; in fact, not a day goes by when you don't learn something new. Sometimes what you learn may take place entirely by sheer chance. Perhaps you listen to the weather forecast and learn the weather prediction for the weekend. You may not even be aware that you have learned something, as very often we do not recognise these informal situations as learning. At other times you may deliberately set out to learn something, for example by joining a workshop on Italian cooking. In these situations you will be aware that you are learning, but because it is for pleasure you may feel differently about this type of learning than previous experiences of formal education. However, no matter what situation you learn in, you will bring to that event your individual learning style.

ACTIVITY 4.1

The point of this activity is to help you understand that learning happens all the time and is based on the experiences that happen to you throughout the day. You don't have to go out of your way to learn something new. The grid below represents the range of different learning opportunities you may encounter, at university and outside, both consciously and unconsciously, in the course of each day. Now think about the types of learning you have done over the last week, and where and how this has taken place. Use the grid to record some examples of different learning experiences you have had. There is an example in each category to get you started.

Conscious learning at university	Unconscious learning at university
• I learned how to take a patient's blood pressure.	• I learned that the lift in B block doesn't stop on the seventh floor.
Conscious learning at home and socially	**Unconscious learning at home and socially**
• I learned how to burn a CD on my laptop.	• I learned that orchids will die if they are overwatered.

Source: Adapted from Honey and Mumford (1989, p1).

Take some time to look at the different learning experiences that you have noted in Activity 4.1. It should be obvious that most of the learning that you do comes directly from your experiences. Sometimes your experiences may be purely accidental and unconscious; however, this does not mean that learning through these experiences is any less valid than deliberate, conscious learning (Honey and Mumford, 1989).

Choosing your learning experiences

It is human nature to gravitate towards experiences that you enjoy, and avoid experiences that you do not enjoy. During your practice placements you will be presented with a range of potential learning experiences, for example practical activities, observation of role models or interacting with people (Harvey and Vaughan, 1990). The point is that you will have a natural tendency towards filtering the range of potential learning opportunities, selecting those that you enjoy and avoiding those that you dislike. As the majority of learning comes through experiences, what and how you learn is largely dependent on the experiences that you choose to engage with. This is particularly true of the unconscious, accidental learning that you do. As a result, your personal likes and dislikes will have a significant impact on the learning experiences available to you.

SCENARIO

Geri lives in London and often drives to Dorset to visit her niece. Geri dislikes driving on major roads as she was involved in a serious motorway accident just after receiving her licence. She prefers to travel on A and B roads for the journey, even though it takes her a little longer. Over the years Geri has worked out her favourite routes, and she now looks forward to travelling through all the different villages and stopping for lunch in a pub along the way. She even allows more time, so that she can make a detour to a farm shop that sells her favourite homemade boysenberry cheesecake. Geri has become a very experienced country driver and has learned a range of alternative routes she can take if there are traffic delays. Geri did not plan to learn these skills; they simply developed as a result of her choices and the experiences she has had.

Understanding your own learning style

The best way to make the most of all potential learning opportunities available to you is to understand your own particular learning style. An appreciation of what makes you 'tick' and the diversity of learning styles among individuals can be the first step towards understanding what types of learning situations will work best for you (McMillan and Dwyer, 1990). It may even explain why you have either consciously or unconsciously chosen or rejected previous experiences. Kolb (1984) suggests that there is a strong relationship between how people learn and how they respond to life situations. It is, therefore, important to recognise your own personality traits and how they contribute to your unique learning style.

Different learning styles

There is a vast range of personality and learning style tests that can help you to understand your own particular style of learning. Before you start this process of discovery, it is important to recognise that no one learning style is any better or worse than any other. There are no right or wrong answers here. There is also a wide range of tests that explore learning styles. The majority of these tests come in questionnaire form and are quite easy to complete. Some tests use personality traits to measure learning preferences. The Myers-Briggs type indicator is one such test (Myers et al., 1998) and discusses four different dichotomies of personality in relation to learning style. Myers (1995) suggests that understanding a student's learning preference can explain why a learner may enjoy and do well at a particular activity. Logic would suggest that the existence of certain personality traits may also explain why a student avoids or does not do well at the opposite types of learning activities.

Other learning style tests are more focused on particular attributes of learning rather than broader determinants of personality, although where one begins and the other ends is almost impossible to unravel. The Learning Styles Questionnaire, developed by Honey and Mumford (1992), is one such tool that can be used for identifying your learning style. The four different learning styles explain not only a preference for a style of learning, but also personality traits that explain preferences for certain experiences over others. It is worth looking at each of the different styles as you may recognise some attributes to be an accurate description of you – both your likes and your dislikes.

HONEY AND MUMFORD LEARNING STYLES

Activists

Activists involve themselves fully and without bias in new experiences. They enjoy the here and now and are happy to be dominated by immediate experiences. They are open-minded, not sceptical, and this tends to make them enthusiastic about anything new. Their philosophy is 'I'll try anything once.' They tend to act first and consider the consequences afterwards. Their days are filled with activity. They tackle problems by brainstorming. As soon as the excitement from one activity has died down, they are busy looking for the next. They tend to thrive on the challenge of new experiences but are bored with implementation and longer term consolidation. They are gregarious people constantly involving themselves with others but, in doing so, they seek to centre all activities around themselves.

Reflectors

Reflectors like to stand back and ponder experiences and observe them from many different perspectives. They collect data, both first hand and from others, and prefer to think about it thoroughly before coming to any conclusion. The thorough collection and analysis of data about experiences and events is what counts so they tend to postpone reaching definitive conclusions for as long as possible. Their philosophy is to be cautious. They are thoughtful people who like to consider all possible angles and implications before making a move. They prefer to take a back seat in meetings and discussions. They enjoy observing other people in action. They listen to others and get the drift of the discussion before making their own points. They tend to adopt a low profile and tend to have a slightly distant, tolerant, unruffled air about them. When they act it is part of a wide picture which includes the past as well as the present and others' observations as well as their own.

Theorists

Theorists adapt and integrate observations into complex but logically sound theories. They think through problems in a vertical, step by step logical way. They assimilate disparate facts into coherent theories. They tend to be perfectionists who won't rest easy until things are tidy and fit into a rational scheme. They like to analyse and synthesise. They are keen on basic assumptions, principles, theories, models and systems thinking. Their philosophy prizes rationality and logic. 'If it's logical it's good.' Questions they frequently ask are: 'Does it make sense?' 'How does this fit with that?' 'What are the basic assumptions?' They tend to be detached, analytical and dedicated to rational objectivity rather than anything subjective or ambiguous. Their approach to problems is constantly logical. This is their 'mental set' and they rigidly reject anything that doesn't fit with it. They prefer to maximise certainty and feel uncomfortable with subjective judgements, lateral thinking and anything flippant.

Pragmatists

Pragmatists are keen on trying out ideas, theories and techniques to see if they work in practice. They positively search out new ideas and take the first opportunity to experiment with applications. They are the sort of people who return from management courses brimming with new ideas that they want to try out in practice. They want to get on with things and act quickly and confidently on ideas that attract them. They tend to be impatient with ruminating and open-ended discussions. They are essentially practical, down to earth people who like making practical decisions and solving problems. They respond to problems and opportunities 'as a challenge'. Their philosophy is: 'There is always a better way' and 'If it works it's good.'

(Honey and Mumford, 1992, pp5–6)

What's my style?

No doubt you will have indentified that you possess certain characteristics of all learning styles; however, there may be one particular style that describes you best. It is quite common to have several attributes of a particular learning style for which you have a strong preference and, conversely, few attributes of a learning style with which you feel less comfortable. As your learning style has quite a lot to do with your personality, you will no doubt see similarities between your learning style and your general likes and dislikes in life.

ACTIVITY 4.2

Take the time now to list your learning styles in order – from what you feel is the most like you, to the style that you feel is least like you.

The learning style that is most like me	
The learning style that is somewhat like me	
The learning style that is a little like me	
The learning style that is least like me	

Learning and your learning style

While understanding your learning style is an interesting process in itself, it is also invaluable in developing your ability to learn and engage with a wide variety of learning experiences. As we have already discovered, some types of learning experiences are geared towards particular styles of learning, so it is likely that you will gravitate towards learning activities that match with your learning style (Honey and Mumford, 1995).

This is especially important when it comes to learning during practice placement. There will be a wide range of learning experiences available to you during your placement; however, depending on your learning style, you may avoid the types of experiences that do not match your learning style. You may not always be aware that you are doing this, especially if you are in a situation where learning is accidental. In fact, if you always select learning experiences that you naturally enjoy, you will be very unlikely to engage 'accidentally' with learning experiences that you don't enjoy. In other words, if there is a mismatch between the learning experience and your learning style, you are much less likely to learn, as you will be limiting your overall learning opportunities (ibid.).

Does age matter?

We already know that age is no barrier to learning. In fact, older learners form the most rapidly growing segment of the learning population in most Western nations (Delahaye and Ehrich, 2008). While it is generally accepted that older learners may not be as quick to learn as younger learners, Crawford (2004) points out that they more than make up for this through a wealth of experience that supports better reasoning and judgement skills. Thus, while your preferred learning style and the way you learn might change as the years progress, age alone is no barrier to learning.

Learning styles and activities

Table 4.1 represents some of the learning activities or experiences that you may come across during a practice placement. The types of activities are grouped together according to the different learning style profiles they may appeal to.

Table 4.1: Learning styles and activities.

Learning style	Learning activities
Activist	• Care of critically ill patients • Bed management issues • Wound care • Diffusing conflict • Emergency situations
Reflector	• Developing and following protocols • Multidisciplinary team (MDT) meetings • Ward rounds • Record keeping • Handover
Theorist	• Discharge planning • Drug calculations • Use of risk assessment tools • Care planning
Pragmatist	• Airway management • Pre- and post-operative care • Infection control procedures • Medication administration • Referrals to community services

Matching your learning style with opportunities

You can see from Table 4.1 that there will naturally be some activities that may match certain learning styles better than others. However, you should also be able to see that avoiding certain learning activities because they do not match a particular style could be a potential problem. Remember that the NMC has determined the competence level required of you throughout your training and at the point of registration (NMC, 2004, 2007). If you avoid learning situations simply because they do not match your learning style, you may also encounter difficulties in achieving competence.

CASE STUDY 4.1

Abosede and Siobhan are second-year students. They have been on a community practice placement at a health centre for two weeks. Every morning the community nurses meet to discuss the clients they will be treating throughout the day, and to make decisions about new referrals. Abosede has come to dread these meetings. The discussion seems to go on too long and she finds it difficult to pay attention to what everyone is saying. She feels that the meeting is a waste of time as, being an activist, she just wants to get on with delivering patient care. She finds she learns most when she is able to discuss each client's needs with her mentor between each visit. Siobhan enjoys the morning review and always listens attentively. She is a reflector and finds it useful to make notes about each client so she can ask her mentor about the various points that were discussed.

In the third week, Abosede and Siobhan are asked if they would like to take on a small client caseload and they both respond enthusiastically. The following day, at the morning review, Abosede is asked to update the team on her clients. She doesn't know what she is expected to report and her mind goes blank. She feels under enormous pressure as everyone is looking at her expectantly. She does a very quick report but feels terrible as she has left out important information and her mentor has to look through her case notes to update the team. Siobhan is also asked to update the group and uses her notes to structure a very detailed report. All eyes are on her and she feels proud to be able to discuss her clients with the team and participate in care planning. Abosede leaves the meeting feeling very frustrated; she knew all the information but just doesn't understand why her report went so wrong.

You will need to make a concerted effort to engage with all learning opportunities, not only those that you naturally enjoy. The good news is that you can develop skills in your least preferred learning style, although it will take some effort and work on your part. Ideally, you should discuss your learning style with your mentor, looking at the types of activities that you most enjoy and establishing a combination of styles that can be incorporated into your learning (Haidar, 2007). Have a look again at Activity 4.2 on page 43 and the learning style that you have the least preference for. There will be very good reasons why this style of learning does not appeal to you; however, in order to make the most of all learning opportunities that come your way, you will need to develop your skills in utilising the full range of learning styles. A starting point is to understand why all learning styles will be important during your practice experience.

Why do I need to be an activist?

If your least preferred learning style is 'activist', it is likely that you will not enjoy learning when it involves a new experience or where there are fresh problems to solve. This will create some difficulties for you in your nurse training as there will be times when action is required and you will need to 'think on your feet'. For example, emergency situations or rapid changes in a patient's clinical condition will require you to make fast and competent decisions as part of a team. This is not the time to spend time thinking through problems or deliberating over the best course of action. Crucially, a part of your learning will be to demonstrate that you can act and react under pressure.

Why do I need to be a reflector?

If your least preferred learning style is 'reflector', it is likely that you will not enjoy learning experiences that involve observing problems or thinking though previous experiences. You will probably not enjoy investigating different types of research and ideas, and may even feel that these activities are a waste of time. However, to demonstrate competence as a nurse you will need to be aware of best practice guidelines and take time to explore alternatives that support evidence-based practice. For example, new wound care techniques or drug therapies may require changes to your clinical practice.

Why do I need to be a theorist?

If your least preferred learning style is 'theorist', it is likely that you will not enjoy spending time over decisions, or lengthy discussions about the best course of action. You may find attention to detail tedious and become frustrated if you cannot get the answer straightaway. However, such skills are vital for nurses, whether you are required to make a complex drug calculation or read carefully through case notes and previous treatment plans. There will be occasions when you will need to take the time to think through problems carefully before acting.

Why do I need to be a pragmatist?

If your least preferred learning style is 'pragmatist', it is likely that you will not enjoy trying out new techniques, or changing the way you do things. You may not be particularly interested in the consequences of actions or outcomes of events. However, 'pragmatic' skills are essential, as these activities are strongly linked to evidence-based practice and to being able to adapt and change patient-care plans so that the best treatment options are delivered. This could include a range of activities, from monitoring fluid and electrolyte balance to re-evaluating a discharge plan.

Learning styles and competence

The simple fact is that you will need to use a range of learning styles in order to develop the competence required of a registered nurse. It just will not be possible to avoid using the full range of learning styles, as you will miss out on learning experiences that are vital for your professional development. Li et al. (2008) comment that the development of new skills and knowledge requires a variety of teaching methods and also learning strategies. Don't worry too much at this stage if you come across a particular learning style that you may struggle with, as we will be looking at practical solutions later in the book.

CHAPTER SUMMARY

Your learning style is as unique as your personality. The style that you use to learn has been developed and sculpted over many years and will be strongly linked to your personal preferences. You must understand your own learning style in order to gain the most from each learning experience. Of equal importance, however, is the need to understand the style of learning in which you are weak or may choose to avoid. The learning opportunities that will be available to you in practice will require that you develop a range of learning styles and techniques, not just those with which you are comfortable and familiar. Competence as a nurse will require a mix of learning styles, in equal and proportional measure.

KNOWLEDGE REVIEW

Having completed the chapter, how would you now rate your knowledge of the following topics?

	Good	Adequate	Poor
1. How your own learning style fits within your personality.			
2. How to match your learning style with a range of clinical activities that suit your style of learning.			
3. The importance of engaging with all learning styles to develop competence.			

Where you're not confident in your knowledge of a topic, what will you do next?

Further reading

Crawford, D (2004) The role of aging in adult learning: implications for instructors in higher education. *New Horizons for Learning.* Available online at **www.newhorizons.org/lifelong/higher_ed/crawford.htm**.
This is a useful essay that looks at the links between ageing, experience, self-esteem and the ability to learn. The particular needs of adult learners are discussed in terms of course content and design.

Useful websites

www.peterhoney.com/ This website allows you to access a variety of Honey and Mumford learning style questionnaires online; however, you will need to pay for them. There is also the option to buy questionnaires in printed form for individuals and groups.

The internet is awash with different types of learning style questionnaires and the following provide just a small sample of the different options available.

www.learning-styles-online.com/inventory/questions.asp
www.engr.ncsu.edu/learningstyles/ilsweb.html
www.vark-learn.com/english/page.asp?p=questionnaire

5. Preparing for clinical placement

CHAPTER AIMS

The aim of this chapter is to assist you with understanding the specific preparation you will need to undertake prior to the commencement of your practice placement.

After reading this chapter you will be able to:

- identify the key aspects of practice preparation;
- consider the relevance of specific placement preparation in terms of your personal needs;
- plan confidently for your learning experiences.

Introduction: putting clinical placement in perspective

Given that you will spend at least 2,300 hours on practice placements, it is important that you make the most of this time. Preparation for your clinical practice is essential for success. Get your preparation right and each placement could be one of the most rewarding and motivating parts of your training. You will have the opportunity to put your brand new skills into practice and link classroom theories with real patient experiences. However, get your preparation wrong and your clinical placements can quickly become times of misery and anxiety. Not only will you become easily discouraged, but you may also jeopardise your performance for practice assessment. The great news is that you can take a great deal of the stress and anxiety out of practice placement simply by preparing yourself for the experience.

Throughout this chapter you will have the opportunity to investigate the essentials of practice preparation. We will start by looking at the major concerns related to clinical placement and how to prepare yourself and plan for a learning experience rather than a working experience. The role of your mentor will also be considered. We will then look at the importance of practical aspects of preparation, such as travel arrangements and juggling other work commitments. The chapter will conclude with a practice placement checklist and an opportunity to consider solutions to problems you may encounter.

Feelings prior to clinical placement

If you are feeling particularly anxious or concerned about your placement, rest assured that this is normal, as even students who appear calm and confident may be feeling very nervous on the inside. You have every right to feel this way because many things will be out of your control while in the practice setting. Sometimes this lack of control and fear of the unknown can lead to high levels of fear and anxiety, especially before a practice placement begins (Beck, 1993). One of the key aspects of preparing for clinical placement is to acknowledge what worries you the most. You may be concerned about whether you will like the clinical area, or if the staff will like you. Having these fears and concerns is totally reasonable, as the clinical environment can be an incredible mix of unpredictable, uncontrollable, challenging and stressful situations (Yong, 1996). A starting point, therefore, is to find out what it is that concerns you. Once you have acknowledged what your fears are, you can start to plan for how you will deal with these situations if they arise.

ACTIVITY 5.1

This list includes some of the typical feelings that past students have felt before their practice placements. You might find it useful to put a tick next to the ones that apply to you. There are some blank boxes in which you might like to write any other feelings you have.

I'm worried that . . .

I won't fit in.	
the people I meet might think I'm stupid.	
it will feel like I'm being thrown in at the deep end.	
I might seem too slow.	
I won't like my mentor, or they won't like me.	
too much might be expected of me.	
I won't get a chance to practise my skills.	
I won't remember everything.	
I might get left alone with a patient and won't know what to do.	
I might hurt someone.	

Take some time now to look at what your main concerns are.

- Is there anything that you are particularly worried about?
- Are your concerns based on a previous experience, or not related to anything in particular?

You may like to make a quick note as to why you are feeling this way, as we will refer back to this list at the end of the chapter.

Preparing for success

If you are preparing for clinical placement for the very first time, there is no doubt that this is a momentous event. Students just like you have described their feelings in the time leading up to their first practice placement as a mix of excitement, fear and ambivalence (Gray and Smith, 1999). Some of these feelings can be attributed to fear of the unknown and anticipatory anxiety (Davies et al., 1994; Gray and Smith, 1999). What you may not realise is that these feelings are perfectly natural, given the fact that you are about to embark on one of the biggest aspects of your nurse training. In fact, Kelly et al. (2007) say that you should expect to feel unsure of how to act and what to do, even if you have practised skills in a previous area.

For obvious reasons, your very first practice placement is likely to be quite daunting, but most students continue to feel nervous prior to all their practice placements. There will be new people to meet, a new environment to discover and a new set of learning objectives to achieve, so it is very important to acknowledge that, every time you embark on a practice placement, you will need to spend some time preparing for the experience. If you do take responsibility and plan for what you can control about your clinical placement, fear of the unknown can be significantly reduced.

Why can't I just turn up on placement?

It is sometimes difficult to understand why you need to prepare for all your practice placements, especially if you have some prior experience to rely on. Spending time on preparation may even seem irrelevant when compared to all the other pressures of your training. It may also be tempting to skip your practice preparation if it is not included as an essential part of your coursework. When the pressures of theoretical work and exams are looming, practice preparation may just seem to be too much effort. Therefore, in order to put the whole issue of practice preparation into perspective, it is important to understand the impact preparation has on your placement as a whole.

Karen and Emma are going on holiday to a wonderful new beach resort in a foreign country. Neither of them has been to the country before, but they have a few weeks before departure to prepare for the trip. Karen starts preparing straightaway. She looks up the resort on the internet and prints out a map of the local area and transport links to and from the airport. She organises some foreign currency, and makes sure her dachshund can be looked after while she is away. Three days before the trip she packs her bag and makes sure her passport and tickets are to hand. On the day of the trip she sets out early for the airport to allow for traffic delays. Karen checks in for her flight and settles down in the departure lounge.

Emma leaves her preparation to the night before as she likes to be more spontaneous. She searches for five hours for her passport and in all the rush forgets to pack her sunglasses and swimsuit. On the trip to the airport she is caught up in traffic delays and has no time to buy her foreign currency before boarding the plane.

Karen enjoys her flight; she thumbs through her travel guide and plans some interesting day trips. Emma spends the flight worrying about how to exchange her money at the destination as she has heard that commission rates are very high.

Karen's first day on holiday is everything she has imagined; she spends her time relaxing on the beach, sipping cocktails and meeting new people. Emma spends her first day rushing about trying to buy a swimsuit and sunglasses. She wastes valuable spending money on an overpriced bikini and worries about how she will afford the rest of her trip.

Be prepared

Being prepared for an event can prevent problems and reduce overall anxiety. The simple fact is that, if you put some time and effort into preparing for placement properly, this will pay dividends when you get there. If you don't prepare for placement, you may find your learning experience less enjoyable and the placement as a whole far more difficult. The good news is that there are many things you can do to improve the experiences that you have on clinical placement before you even get there. However, you will need to accept that you are responsible for your own practice preparation. Either you decide to do it or you don't. No one can prepare you for your experience apart from you.

Planning for learning success

Before you even contemplate setting foot in your next clinical placement, you will need to plan for how you are going to learn. Some students make the big mistake of thinking that learning will just naturally happen once they turn up on the placement. Kelly et al. (2007) term this a 'doing' attitude, where students rush into a clinical placement with a big list of what they need to 'do', rather than what they need to 'learn'. In this case, many students will return from a placement saying that they didn't learn anything (Elcock, 2006). This attitude can also result in a student feeling as if they are being used as an extra pair of hands, rather than being treated as a learner.

It is vitally important, therefore, that you enter the clinical environment with an understanding of what you need to learn while you are there, and how you plan to do it. This will assist you to remain focused on these objectives from the very beginning. Elcock et al. (2007) argue that it is all too easy for mentors to mistake your participation in practice as a contribution to their work rather than your learning opportunity. This is far from the ideal situation, and it is easy to want to blame your mentor for this. However, if you think about it logically, you will realise that your mentor is not entirely responsible for your learning. Unless you know why you are there and what you should be doing, your mentor may just accept a situation in which you are helping to get the work done (Elcock, 2006).

Planning your learning outcomes

You must, therefore, enter your clinical placement with a mindset as a 'learner' rather than a 'doer'. This means that you will need to review all your learning outcomes prior to your placement and start planning for how you will achieve these. The earlier you start preparing, the better; and leaving your preparation until the night before is hardly ideal.

Therefore, before your clinical placement starts you should review your learning outcomes and draw up a list of everything you need to learn while you are there (Elcock, 2006). Not only will this help to keep you focused on what you need to learn, but it will make a great first impression when you meet your mentor. It will also help to clarify with your mentor that you are there to learn *through* doing, not just there to *do*.

Learning outcomes and learning opportunities

The first step is to start matching up your learning outcomes with learning opportunities – actually quite a simple process. Begin by making a list of the different learning outcomes you will be required to achieve on the placement; that is, a list of what will be expected of you during your placement. Once you have formulated your list, you can then start to plan the types of activities that may be available to you that match up with each learning opportunity. In other words, a list of *how* you plan to achieve the *what*.

ACTIVITY 5.2

The aim of this activity is to improve your awareness of potential learning opportunities in practice placement. The table below provides some examples of learning outcomes matched with learning opportunities. You can see that each outcome is matched to a variety of potential experiences that could be turned into opportunities to learn. Use the blank boxes to draw up your own list, making links between *what* you need to do and *how* you plan to do it. You may like to refer to a previous or current practice assessment booklet to make this activity realistic and relevant to your own experiences.

Learning outcome (What)	Learning opportunity (How)
Communication skills	• Handover of patients • Answering the telephone • Documenting care plans
Medicine administration	• Medication rounds • Preparing IV infusions

Planning through using resources

There may be a number of resources available to you to help with planning your learning opportunities. For example, your university may have information about clinical placements online and, if so, you will have been provided with information on how to access the required websites during your programme. If this resource is available to you, it is to your advantage to look at any placement information and complete any suggested preparation. Online resources often provide additional information to help with planning your learning experiences and what you can expect while you are there. They can be updated more frequently than printed material and, as a result, are a valuable source of information.

It is also likely that you will have been provided with suggested readings or activities to complete prior to undertaking your clinical experience. In addition, you may be required to complete preparatory work in your assessment document before the placement begins. These may be e-learning activities, or presented to you in the form of classroom discussion or a workbook. It is quite possible that some of this work may be self-directed in nature and not directly linked to your assessment criteria. If this is the case, the temptation not to engage with preparatory work can be quite high.

It is common for students to dedicate the majority of their time to activities for which there are marks to be earned. It may also be difficult for you to see the relevance of the suggested readings to your next clinical placement (Wilkinson et al., 1998). However, specific pre-placement preparation is there to assist you in gaining independence in your practice learning. The more independent you are, the more you will enjoy your placement, as you will be given greater responsibility and have more opportunities to practise different tasks (Lofmark and Wikblad, 2001). If there is specific placement preparation recommended to you, you should definitely undertake this.

Understanding where you are going

It is really important that you understand the nature of the clinical area to which you will be going for your placement. Turning up on your first day without knowing about the specialty area is a major mistake, and is actually quite insulting to the placement area concerned. It will be noticed if you have taken the time to undertake preparatory research in the specialty, as this will be reflected in the questions that you ask while on placement (Sharples, 2007a). Not only will the lack of preparation impact on your learning experience, but your mentor may interpret this as a lack of interest in the placement. Inadequate preparation may result in a negative first impression of you and make it more difficult for you to fit into the clinical environment (Fitzpatrick et al., 1996). Once again, there may be websites that you can access with this sort of information, and your university may have specific practice placement information available for you to access.

CASE STUDY 5.1

A mentor speaks about the frustration of having a student come into the placement area without making an effort to prepare:

We had this student a few months ago who just turned up on his first day and right from the start it was obvious he didn't have a clue what we do here. We're an orthopaedic ward, and he's just standing there looking blank and it was pretty obvious he didn't know what the word 'orthopaedic' meant. He may as well have hung a big sign around his neck that said, 'I don't want to be here', as far as I was concerned. It was just so frustrating, for him and for us, because we just don't have

> *time here to spend hours explaining the basic stuff that students should already know. If he had put the effort into us, then no problem, we would have put the effort into him. In the end it took him about two weeks to catch on and by that time he'd missed out on so much the whole thing was a bit of a waste really.*

Planning a visit

In most cases you will find it useful to arrange a pre-placement visit as part of your preparation. It is never a good idea to turn up unannounced, so make a phone call to find out if a visit is suitable for the clinical area, and to arrange a good day and time. You may have an opportunity to meet key staff before your placement starts and familiarise yourself with the layout of the workplace (Sharples, 2007a). This is also a great way to introduce yourself to your mentor. All of this can help to reduce your pre-placement anxiety. Such a visit can also be a good way to plan for the learning opportunities available to you, as you may be able to ask more questions about the specialty. If your approach is right, it can also make a great first impression, as you will come across as keen, eager and prepared to learn.

Practical planning

Plan your travel

Obviously, you want to create the very best first impression when you turn up for placement on the first day, and turning up on time in the correct location is one of the best ways to do this. One of the easiest and least complicated aspects of preparing for a practice placement is planning how you will travel to and from your clinical area. This may seem a little obvious, but placements will be in many different types of location, and often students have been caught out by this aspect, even those who have prepared thoroughly in other ways. If you have prepared for this, you will have more time to devote to learning and less to worrying about being late.

TOP TIPS FOR PLANNING TRAVEL

- Use a map to plan your journey to avoid getting lost and carry the map with you.
- If you are using public transport, check travel times for all your different shifts.
- Have a contingency plan for weekends and public holidays as your travel time may be longer or shorter than usual.

- If you are planning on driving or cycling, find out where you can park your car or bike safely for the duration of the shift.
- Find out the cost of parking meters and carry change if necessary.
- Consider a 'trial run' well in advance of your first day so you know what to expect during the journey and when you arrive.
- Use the resources your university has for planning journeys to clinical placements, or online journey planners.
- Add some additional time to your planned journey to allow for last-minute problems, for example traffic delays.

Life outside clinical placement

On every single clinical placement that you undertake, you will need to consider how you are going to cope with and manage your life outside. Once again, you may be able to predict some events and to plan before the placement how to manage these situations when they arise.

Shift work

Without any doubt, your clinical placement will impact significantly on your home and family life. Shift work and the requirement for you to work alongside your mentor will result in the need for you to do unsocial hours that may not fit in with current childcare arrangements and social or work commitments. Unfortunately, some students make the mistake of thinking that, once they have informed the placement of their special circumstances, adjustments will be made to their off-duty hours to accommodate their needs (Sharples, 2006). This is not the case and you should certainly not expect it. It is essential, therefore, that you make adequate arrangements before your placement commences so that your personal life does not impact on your availability for clinical practice. The NMC makes your position, and your mentor's, very clear on this issue: *Whilst giving direct care in the practice setting at least 40 per cent of a student's time must be spent being supervised (directly or indirectly) by a mentor* (2008, p30).

The meaning of this directive is very clear. Every time you are involved in direct patient care during your clinical placement, a mentor is required to supervise you. Therefore, the onus is on you to be available to fit in with your mentor's rota and this leaves very limited options for negotiating your own shift pattern. Combine this directive with the NMC requirement that students must be exposed to the full range of 24-hour/7 days a week care in relation to practice experience (NMC, 2004) and it becomes very clear that family-friendly hours are not going to be a part of your life as a student. You will need to plan for how to cope with this prior to clinical placement.

Part-time work

Many students find that the difficulty of juggling part-time work commitments around clinical practice causes them considerable stress. As a result of the NMC regulations, it is impossible to have any sort of fixed work commitment as, sooner or later, it will clash with your practice experience. While there is no problem with you having a job while you are undertaking your nursing course, any employment must be flexible around your practice placement, not the other way round. The same goes for the theory part of the programme. In other words, you will need to arrange your life to meet the requirements of the nursing programme; the programme cannot be altered to suit you. For this reason, your best option for part-time work would be casual employment, perhaps as part of a nursing bank or agency.

Smoking

If you are a smoker, you will need to plan for how to cope with this during your clinical placement. The days of smoking in tearooms and designated smoking areas are long gone, so a quick cigarette break while on placement is out of the question. Depending on your placement area, it may just not be possible to go outside for a cigarette, and a smoking break may make you unpopular and have an impact on your learning opportunities (Elcock, 2007). Your options are to consider giving up smoking prior to placement, or to plan for some type of nicotine replacement that will curb your cravings. Whatever you decide to do is up to you; the most important thing is that you do have a plan of how to cope. This may seem trivial; however, for many students this can affect their enjoyment and commitment to placement.

Sickness and absences

Obviously, some events are unpredictable and cannot always be specifically planned for. However, you can plan ahead for what you will do when unpredictable events do occur. For example, sickness and burst water pipes can all happen with very little warning, but may result in you being unable to attend placement. You will therefore need to have contact details available of relevant people whom you may need to inform if you cannot attend clinical placement. Extended periods of absence will have an impact on your learning opportunities, so you should make yourself aware of relevant policies before the placement commences. At the very least, you should review your student policy on sickness and absence, as this will provide information on what to do and whom to contact, and check the policy on make-up time, to provide support for you should you need it.

Final preparation

Before you embark on your practice placement, the final step is to make sure absolutely everything you need to do and plan for is in order. Remember that, the more you plan, the less likely it is that you will encounter unpredictable events.

ACTIVITY 5.3

Use this check list to ensure that you really are prepared for all aspects of your practice placement. Put a tick next to each of the elements that applies to you.

I know where I am going on clinical placement.	
I have organised my travel arrangements.	
I have reviewed my learning outcomes.	
I have matched my learning outcomes with learning opportunities.	
I have arranged a pre-placement visit.	
I have the contact numbers and details of where I am going.	
I have done the preparation work recommended to me.	
I have looked at the website for placement information (if available).	
I know exactly where to go and whom to ask for when I get there.	
I am available for the full range of shifts that I might be required to do.	
I have reviewed my university policies on sickness and make-up time.	
I have the contact details of lecturers I may need to call while on placement.	
I know whom to contact if I cannot attend placement.	
I have planned how to cope with my nicotine cravings (if required).	
I have a uniform or appropriate clothes as required.	
I have completed the relevant sections of my practice assessment document.	

Now refer back to Activity 5.1 to see what aspects of practice placement you were concerned about when we began this chapter. If you are able to tick each box confidently in the checklist, it is very likely that your original fears have been well and truly dealt with. In most cases, your original fears were related to fear of the unknown, and preparation for clinical placement allows you to confront and deal with this.

Problems and solutions

It may be that, despite working through the checklist, you still have some areas of concern that have not been resolved. If this is the case, you must resolve these issues before the placement begins. You will need to identify exactly what your concerns are in order to find a solution. Identifying any likely problems and what you can actively do about these issues will help you to feel more in control of your clinical placement and more confident regarding your performance as a whole.

ACTIVITY 5.4

Use the following table to write down any concerns you may have regarding your upcoming clinical placement. Next to each problem write down what you feel the solution might be. Try to be as systematic as possible as problems are best dealt with step by step. Once you have decided upon a possible solution it is up to you to make this happen.

Pre-placement concerns	Solutions

CHAPTER SUMMARY

In this chapter we have discussed the importance of preparing for practice placement and how thorough preparation can improve your overall learning experience. Understanding what, how and when to prepare for your practice experience is vital in terms of reducing your anxiety and making the most of all learning opportunities that may come your way. The choice regarding how much or little you do in terms of your practice preparation is down to you, and it will require a certain amount of self-direction and intrinsic motivation (see Chapter 9). However, while there will be some effort required, it will not go to waste and, ultimately, you will be the one to reap the rewards.

KNOWLEDGE REVIEW

Having completed the chapter, how would you now rate your knowledge of the following topics?

	Good	Adequate	Poor
1. The key aspects of practice preparation.			
2. The relevance of specific placement preparation in terms of your personal needs.			
3. How to plan confidently for your learning experiences.			

Where you're not confident in your knowledge of a topic, what will you do next?

Further reading

Elcock, K (2006) Wake up and learn. *Nursing Standard*, 20(49): 61.
A short article that provides insight into student experiences on practice placement.

Useful website

www.rcn.org.uk/__data/assets/pdf_file/0011/78545/001815.pdf
This toolkit, entitled 'Helping students get the most from their practice placements', provides an overview of the student role and responsibilities while on placement. There is a small section on student responsibility in relation to practice preparation.

6. Self-regulated learning in practice

CHAPTER AIMS

The aim of this chapter is to provide an understanding of the theory behind, and purpose of, self-regulated learning in practice.

After reading this chapter you will be able to:

- understand the main principles of self-regulated learning and the specific challenges of learning in practice;

- appreciate the importance of self-regulated learning skills in developing your competence;

- recognise the role of your mentor in facilitating self-regulated learning.

Introduction: self-regulated learning – setting the scene

In the previous chapter, we discussed the need to prepare for your clinical placement in order to obtain maximum benefit from all your learning experiences. We now know that the **motivation** to prepare for clinical placement is largely dependent on the ability to learn as an adult, and involves the skill of self-regulated learning. However, the ability to be a self-regulated learner is important not only for placement preparation; it is also a vital skill to master in order to create the best possible learning opportunities during the actual placement. Without this skill you could find yourself struggling to cope with the practice elements of your course, as these will have been designed for an adult learner.

The focus of this chapter will be on exploring the nature of self-regulation skills in relation to practice, and ways in which these skills can be developed to your advantage. The starting point is to define 'self-regulation' and how this is applicable to the practice learning environment. There will be an opportunity to investigate the particular challenges of practice learning, and how to be a self-regulated learner to meet these challenges. We will then consider the importance of self-regulated learning in terms of the professional competencies expected of you as a nurse, and the role of your mentor in relation to self-regulation. In addition, you will be able to identify how your pre-existing skills can be developed into self-regulatory learning skills.

Self-regulated learning

Self-regulation is fundamentally a state of being, rather than a state of doing. While **self-direction** involves the function of organising your learning, self-regulated learning is focused on using your own motivation and drive to develop your own learning experience. Sung (2006) explains that self-regulated learners set their own task-specific learning goals and employ appropriate strategies to attain these goals. These may be very different from the self-directed activities you may have already engaged in, where the learning goal may have been given to you. These may include self-study days or activities such as problem-based learning, blended learning, clinical learning logs or independent learning contracts (Smedley, 2007). In fact, study for exams or assignment preparation may also be classed as a self-directed activity.

In this context, 'self-direction' is a euphemism for undertaking a task or activity with minimum supervision. While such a skill is commendable, it is important to recognise that there is a clear distinction between *doing* a self-directed activity, and *being* a self-regulated learner. While the difference may appear subtle, in reality they are worlds apart. It is important to recognise that gaining the most from your practice learning opportunities will require you to develop and master the skills of self-regulated learning.

Learning in theory, learning in practice

It is not uncommon for students to put a great deal of effort into addressing academic challenges, assuming that the skills they attain while undertaking the theory programme will readily transfer to the clinical environment. However, the challenges of the clinical environment are very different from the types of issues you may encounter during your theory work. These different challenges mean that you will need to develop a new range of skills to cope with and learn during practice. You will essentially be required to demonstrate competence in a wide range of areas, such as knowledge development, critical understanding, practical skills and professional values and standards (Flanagan et al., 2000). In Chapter 3 (Figure 3.1, page 32) we identified that learning in practice requires the ability to apply, under supervision, a combination of cognitive, psychomotor and affective skills to solve problems and make clinical decisions (Windsor, 1987). On Figure 3.1, these three aspects of competence were termed 'knowledge', 'skills' and 'professionalism'. So the skills that you will need for learning in practice will be vastly different from the skills you may have developed during theoretical coursework.

ACTIVITY 6.1

We already know that learning in theory is different from learning in practice. If you have already been on a practice placement, you will be familiar with some of the differences. Use this table to note down the different challenges you have already faced or think you may face during clinical placement as opposed to the theoretical part of your course. Try to think specifically about the skills you may need for each environment and how these may differ. An example has been provided to get you started.

Current skills in theory learning	Challenges of clinical learning
Presenting information during a tutorial session to classmates I know well.	Presenting information during a team meeting to clinical staff I don't know at all.

Take some time to reflect on the list you have compiled in Activity 6.1, as some of the challenges for practice learning may be quite surprising. Just because you are confident in one skill in theory does not mean you will be able to transfer the same confidence to practice. The good news is that, once you understand your learning needs, you can learn how to transfer your skills to cope with these challenges.

Learning to be self-regulated

We spend our whole lives learning new skills and putting these skills into practice in order to function normally. In fact, we have learned so many skills during the course of our lifetimes that we take many of them for granted. We use some skills so often during the course of a normal day that we don't even think consciously about the skill at all while we are using it. For example, you are reading this book, and reading is a pretty amazing skill. You had to be taught how to read, and at first this was probably quite difficult as you learned all the different letters and sounds. However, now that you have learned to read, it is unlikely that you think about the process at all, as it just becomes an automatic part of your life.

ACTIVITY 6.2

Stop for a minute and think about all the times today when you used your reading skills, then use the box below to make a list.

> The ways I have used my reading skills today include . . .

You may have had to think hard about the list you compiled in Activity 6.2, and no doubt you have probably forgotten to include quite a few obvious situations. For example, did you remember to include reading the message board on your fridge door, or the name of the cheese you sliced for your sandwich? What about the street sign you drove past, or when you updated your profile on 'Facebook'? The truth is that you are able to use your reading skills all day every day without consciously thinking about them. You have learned how to transfer your reading skills into a wide range of different situations.

Low-road transfer

When skills that you have developed become automatic and part of your subconscious, this is referred to as **low-road transfer**, (Salomon and Perkins, 1989). Using low-road transfer you are able to apply your skills with very little in the way of mindfulness or conscious deliberation (Sung, 2006). In other words, you are able to do something without having to think about it. Have a look again at the list you created in Activity 6.2 regarding the times you used your reading skills today. Now imagine if you had to think about how to use your reading skills every single time you needed to read. No doubt you would be quite frustrated, and may have missed out on some important events. The point is that the ability to employ low-road transfer actually helps in adapting and functioning quickly within a variety of situations without getting bogged down in detail or needing to analyse each separate event. The main benefit of low-road transfer is that the more varied the situations in which you utilise a certain skill, the more automatic the application becomes (Sung, 2006). Therefore, while you may have learned to read using books, you can adapt this same skill to reading anything at all without needing consciously to think about it.

High-road transfer

Of course, the opposite of low-road transfer is **high-road transfer**. Salomon and Perkins (1989) describe high-road transfer as a way of examining a situation, then deciding on an alternative action when faced with an infamiliar task. For example, while you might use low-road transfer to read a book, you will need high-road transfer to understand and make sense of what you are reading. The fact is that you will have to employ high-road transfer skills in order to become a self-regulated learner in practice. While low-road transfer skills are primarily focused on getting the job done, high-road transfer skills allow you to question why you are doing the job. In order to be a self-regulated learner you must strive to develop and maintain a high-road transfer approach within your learning experience. While low-road transfer may help you to perform a task adequately, high-road transfer will prompt you to question why you are performing the task. In other words, while low-road transfer is about doing, high-road transfer is about knowing why you do.

CASE STUDY 6.1

Dev is a second-year student undertaking his clinical placement on an acute surgical ward. One of his objectives on the placement was to demonstrate competence in administering subcutaneous injections. Every day he has had the opportunity to undertake this skill and his mentor has indicated that he is competent with his injection technique. Dev has become so confident that he does not really think about the task any more, as it has become routine.

One morning, Dev is being supervised by his mentor on the medication round and begins to prepare a subcutaneous injection for his patient. His mentor stops him and enquires about the patient's latest blood results. Dev has not thought to look at the results; he has been so focused on performing the task that he has not checked to see if the medication should be given. The patient's blood results are checked and it becomes clear that the injection is no longer required. If Dev had preceded with the injection, this would have resulted in a serious drug error. It becomes clear to Dev and his mentor that, while he may have learned to perform an injection competently, he does not have the skill of managing the safe care of his patient.

High-road transfer and self-regulation

From the above, we can see that there is a very strong link between high-road transfer and self-regulation. If you adopt low-road transfer on your clinical placements, your learning experience will become a sequence of tasks and activities that you move from and to with little understanding of why you are performing the tasks, or the significance of those tasks. Even worse, your learning will be dictated by the availability of tasks, and when these specific activities are not supplied, you may find yourself at a loss and feeling as if you do not know what to do. This is because you see your role as a doer, rather than a knowledgeable doer. So high-road transfer is vital because it allows you to comprehend the appropriateness of applying a previously acquired skill in an entirely new situation (Sung, 2006). It will be your ability to utilise high-road transfer that will provide opportunities for demonstrating your competence within the unpredictability of the clinical environment. Sung (2006) argues that your ability to use conscious deliberation with only limited guidance is more likely to produce real understanding, rather than the formulaic learning that results from repetition and extended practice.

Self-regulation and the NMC

The NMC makes it very clear that the requirement for nurses to be self-regulated in their practice is not negotiable. Among other requirements, in order to achieve fitness for practice, a registered nurse must demonstrate the ability to search the evidence base, disseminate research findings and adapt practice where necessary (NMC, 2004). These requirements are entirely self-regulatory and are implicit within the domain of professional accountability and responsibility. As a consequence, Zimmerman (1995) highlights that self-regulated learning encapsulates three distinct phases: planning, performance and evaluation. It is no coincidence that such skills are synonymous with the need to reflect on practice that is required for safe and competent care within a work-based learning context (Flanagan et al., 2000). These are also the skills related to high-road transfer. Reflection on practice does not fit with a low-road transfer approach. You will need to be self-regulated in order to demonstrate your competence for qualification.

Self-regulation and your mentor

Many students return from their clinical placements disappointed with the experience and feeling as if they have learned nothing (Elcock, 2006). It is not uncommon for students to feel as if they are being used as 'just a pair of hands', blaming their mentors for limited learning experiences. There are some very important issues here, but it is important to get one point clear right from the start. As we discussed in Chapter 3, your mentor does not have sole responsibility or accountability for your learning. This is a shared experience, so you should be prepared to regulate your own learning experiences.

The fact is that some students do not take advantage of all potential learning experiences as they are waiting to be told what to do, either by their mentor or through information provided by the university. However, your mentor is only required to *provide* a learning experience and opportunity for you. If you do not take advantage of the experiences and opportunities available to you, this is not your mentor's fault. In terms of your learning experiences, as long as your mentor is fulfilling their role in relation to the *Standards for Learning and Assessment in Practice* (NMC, 2008), the rest is up to you.

CASE STUDY 6.2

A mentor speaks about the pleasure of working with students who demonstrate self-regulation skills:

You can always tell the really keen students. They're the ones that are always asking questions and don't hang around waiting to be told what to do. They get stuck in, and you find that you want to spend more time explaining things because they obviously want to learn and put the effort in themselves. They know what they want to learn, and don't expect me to do the learning for them. I'll go out of my way for these students, because you know they are really trying hard and want to learn as much as possible.

The clinical environment is packed with potential learning opportunities. Virtually every activity that takes place has the potential to be turned into a learning experience. Kelly et al. (2007) recommend that you are up front with your mentor about what you want to learn on your clinical placement, and what you are already competent in doing. It is your awareness and insight into your own learning needs that will form the basis of self-regulation. Therefore, if you show a genuine interest and enthusiasm from the start, this will pay dividends throughout the placement. Remember, though, that you will only be able to speak knowledgeably about your learning objectives if you have prepared thoroughly for practice.

CASE STUDY 6.3

Victoria and Mel are first-year students undertaking their practice placements in a care home. Victoria is having a very unhappy time as she feels she is learning nothing. Every day her mentor allocates her a small group of residents to care for and, although she has been practising skills of personal care and communication, she feels let down that there is not more to learn. She spends a lot of time sitting in the day room looking through patient notes and wishing she was on a better placement. She has asked to leave early several times when she feels that there is nothing to do.

Mel is learning far more than she could have expected. As well as caring for her residents, she makes time every day to participate in the medication round with her mentor, and has been able to learn about the actions of at least three major drug groupings. She has asked to spend a day shadowing the physiotherapist, and has been able to participate in team meetings and lead a therapy group. Every day she sets herself new goals of what she would like to learn and discusses with her mentor how best to meet her goals. Mel feels that everyone is going out of their way to help her. Victoria feels that Mel is getting special treatment and wonders why no one seems interested in her.

Can I be self-regulated?

Your own expectations and experiences on entering the nursing programme will no doubt have some impact on your ability to be a self-regulated learner in practice. Nurse educators also play an important role in assisting students to apply their knowledge in the clinical area (Beck, 1993). It is well recognised that nursing programmes do not always place enough emphasis on skills for self-regulated learning in practice. At the time of writing, there is a call within the nursing literature to provide orientation programmes that focus on the importance of self-regulatory learning strategies for student nurses (Mullen, 2007).

As a direct result, many nursing programmes are providing training for learning in practice. It may be that your current nursing course puts specific emphasis on helping you to develop self-regulation skills for learning in practice. This may even be referred to as 'learning to learn'. If this is the case, you are in a very fortunate position and should make the most of these development opportunities.

However, your ability to self-regulate your learning may also be related to your assumptions about the teaching you expect will be provided during the programme and your role in relation to learning. For example, some nursing students expect that their course will be teacher-directed and tightly structured (MacLeod, 1995). Like many students in the past, you may have entered the nursing course expecting to receive lectures, be provided with course material, involve yourself in some classroom discussion and complete the required assessments and exams (Wilkinson et al., 1998). If these were your expectations, you may have found the transition from being a passive recipient to being an active participant in your own learning quite daunting (Wilkinson et al., 1998). If this is true for you in the theory element of the course, learning in practice will be far more daunting in terms of your self-regulation skills.

Skills for self-regulated learning

You cannot expect to turn into a self-regulated learner overnight. Remember, this is a skill that will take considerable time and effort to master. To become self-regulated during your practice learning experience will require you to consider the types of activities that will be available to you, and also the feasibility of you taking part in these activities. You should also take your preferred learning style into account as well, as this will make the learning experience far more enjoyable. This may sound like a very complicated way to undertake seemingly simple learning experiences, but remember that you are aiming towards high-road transfer skills in order to become a knowledgeable doer. The good news is that self-regulation of learning can be easily mastered and adopted in order to learn through your practice experiences. In the next chapter we will explore how to self-regulate your clinical placement in order to learn in, through and during placement.

CHAPTER SUMMARY

The need to develop the skills of high-road transfer cannot be denied in terms of learning in practice. If you want to become a competent practitioner, you must provide evidence of self-regulated learning ability and such skills cannot be obtained without the use of high-road transfer. There is a clear need, therefore, to develop your skills of self-regulated learning in practice. Once you have developed the skills that support high-road transfer, you will be able to self-regulate your practice learning opportunities. The development of self-regulatory learning skills is the basis for learning in, through and during practice placement.

KNOWLEDGE REVIEW

Having completed the chapter, how would you now rate your knowledge of the following topics?

	Good	Adequate	Poor
1. The main principles of self-regulated learning and the specific challenges of learning in practice.			
2. The importance of self-regulated learning skills in developing your competence.			
3. The role of your mentor in facilitating self-regulated learning.			

Where you're not confident in your knowledge of a topic, what will you do next?

Further reading

Brockett, R and Hiemstra, R (1991) *Self-direction in Adult Learning: Perspectives on research and practice.* London: Routledge.

This book provides useful insight into the theory and research that underpins self-direction in relation to adult learning. The book offers strategies for applying the principles of self-direction and self-regulation in practice.

Useful website

www.health.heacademy.ac.uk/ The Higher Education Academy has a subject centre dedicated to health sciences and practice. Links to the practice education and support special interest group provide valuable information on current research and practices within practice learning environments.

7. Learning through experience

CHAPTER AIMS

The aim of this chapter is for you understand how you can use self-regulation to learn in, through and during your clinical experiences. After reading this chapter you will be able to:

- understand the link between self-regulated learning and learning through experience;

- apply the principles of a learning cycle in order to plan your placement learning experiences;

- identify how you can use reflection to learn from placement experiences.

Introduction: learning to learn in practice

Every time you go on a clinical placement, you will have the opportunity of learning in, through and during a range of practice experiences. The experiences that you may encounter may be planned, foreseeable structured events, or random, coincidental and spontaneous. The nature of the event matters little, as all events, whether predictable or spontaneous, have one essential thing in common – they are all potential learning experiences.

Yet we now know that being provided with opportunities to learn in practice does not automatically mean that learning will take place. Some students make the mistake of thinking that, once they are in practice, learning will just naturally happen. However, after reading the preceding chapters and taking part in the various activities, it should be clear that learning does not just happen; you will have to make it happen. First, you will need to develop the skills of an adult learner (Chapter 2) and, second, you will need to self-regulate your learning experiences (Chapter 6). In addition, any barriers that may impact on your ability to learn must be dealt with, either by removing these barriers or reducing their impact so that you are free to learn.

Therefore, while there are opportunities to learn in practice, it is also important to seek out and use these opportunities. In this chapter we will discover how to do just that. The starting point will be to establish the types of clinical experiences that may be developed into learning experiences. From this point, we will discuss how to use self-regulation to plan and structure learning, using Kolb's experiential learning cycle as an example. As well as exploring how you can learn by using a learning cycle, we will examine how to use reflection as a means of learning during and after clinical experiences. The chapter will conclude by discussing how your learning experience can be designed to match to your individual learning style within a learning cycle.

Learning through clinical experiences

The clinical environment is a never-ending source of potential learning experiences that become more meaningful the more you participate (Andrews and Roberts, 2003). In fact, some experiences are guaranteed to occur every day. For example, if you are on a ward placement in a hospital, you can be certain that there will be medications administered to patients during the course of the shift. Likewise, if you are on a community placement in a day centre, you will have opportunities to communicate with service users. There will also be experiences available that cannot be planned for. For example, a patient you are caring for on a hospital ward may suddenly experience a drop in blood pressure and require urgent treatment. Or a client in a day centre may have a verbal argument with another client and you may need rapidly to diffuse a tense situation. In fact, virtually everything that takes place during your clinical experience can be turned into an opportunity for you to learn.

The challenge is knowing *how* to turn your clinical experiences into learning experiences. Unless you do this, your clinical experiences will become a series of random events and learning opportunities will be wasted. A good starting point is for you to know how to identify the types of experiences, both planned and unplanned, that you may encounter on clinical placement.

ACTIVITY 7.1

Use the grid to make a note of a few different types of experiences that occur during a clinical placement. Pay particular attention to whether the experiences are predictable or unpredictable. There is an example in each column to get you started.

Predictable experiences	Unpredictable experiences
Documenting in client notes	Making changes to a client's care plan following an MDT meeting

Take some time to consider the differences between the two lists you made in Activity 7.1. Did you have difficulty identifying 'unpredictable experiences'? This was not meant to confuse you – it was to demonstrate that it is impossible to predict every experience you will have during a practice placement.

Predictable and unpredictable learning experiences

It should now be very clear that, while practice learning is all about experiences, it is actually impossible to predict a significant percentage of the experiences that you will encounter. The paradox is that a great deal of your learning, and sometimes the best experiences, will take place as a result of unplanned, unexpected, random experiences.

The great news is that it is possible to learn through all experiences whether they are predictable or not. The key is having a plan of how to make the most of all your experiences, both predictable and unpredictable, to ensure that you are able to turn them into learning experiences. You may not be able to plan or predict what will take place in practice; however, you can plan for how you can learn from all experiences that come your way.

Learning through personal experience

Before we go any further, it is important to establish that people experience the same events in different ways. No doubt you have already been in a situation where your experience of an event was the exact opposite of someone else's. Perhaps a guest speaker came along to one of your tutorial sessions. You may have found the speaker wonderful, felt they had a lot of interesting anecdotes on a fascinating topic and were disappointed that the session was limited to one hour. However, someone else in the group may have had exactly the opposite experience; they found the topic dull and the speaker uninspiring. Boud et al. (1993) explain that this happens because the meaning of an experience is not a given, but is subject to interpretation.

ACTIVITY 7.2

Take some time to consider the following statement:

> When different learners are involved in the same event, their experience of it will be different and they will construct and reconstruct it differently. What learners bring to an event – their expectations, knowledge, attitude and emotions – will influence their interpretation of it and their own construction of what they experience. An event can influence a learner but only if the learner is predisposed to being influenced.
>
> (Boud et al., 1993, p11)

Now think about a time in your life when you shared an experience with someone but had a different reaction. You may choose to relate this to a clinical experience, or to something in your personal life.

- Why do you think this happened?
- What factors may have influenced your different reactions?

You may like to make some brief notes about the expectations, knowledge, attitude and emotions that influenced your interpretation of the event.

Making learning personal

What and how you learn from the experiences that you encounter on a clinical placement will be personal to you. The fact that you will be exposed to clinical experiences during your practice placement does not automatically mean that you will learn something as a result of the experience. You must actually *want* to learn something. This means that the difference between an *experience* and a *learning experience* is you. Learning will not happen by osmosis; it starts and ends with you.

In Chapter 6 we indentified this as self-regulated learning. If you have the drive, determination and motivation to learn through all the clinical experiences you encounter, they will become learning experiences. However, if you fail to treat all your experiences as learning opportunities, your placement will mean little to you and countless learning opportunities will be lost. This would be the equivalent of sleepwalking through your placement (Elcock, 2006) – your body may have been there, but your brain has been asleep.

A plan for learning

No learning will happen unless you are clear about what it is you would like to learn. The learning outcomes that you bring to your clinical placement will already supply you with this information. Remember that these learning objectives are derived from the *Standards of Proficiency* (NMC, 2004) and *Essential Skills Clusters* (NMC, 2007) documents. This means that what you need to learn is based on what the NMC requires you to learn, so this needs to be taken very seriously. Understanding what you are required to learn should form part of your preparation for your practice placement and the whole of Chapter 5 was dedicated to this theme. If you really want to learn in practice, thorough preparation before you arrive is essential.

CASE STUDY 7.1

Ann is a second-year student and has been allocated a practice placement in an oncology day care clinic. In preparation for placement, Ann reads through the ten learning objectives in her practice assessment document. One of her learning objectives reads as follows:

Learning Outcome 7

Demonstrate sensitivity to the diverse care needs of patients and clients when planning and managing care.

In the weeks leading up to the placement, Ann puts some time into her practice preparation. Her university has a practice education website, and she makes a point of working through the online pre-placement activities and also visits the clinic to introduce herself to the staff working there. She realises that she will be caring for a wide age range of patients and looks forward to this challenge. Ann arrives for her first day of clinical placement ready to learn.

Experiential learning

When you arrive on practice placement you should have already planned, and be clear about, *what* you want to learn, as did Ann in Case study 7.1. However, you also need to plan *how* you are going to learn. While we have already seen in Chapter 6 that self-regulation is essential for learning in, through and during practice, without a clear plan of *how* to do this, learning experiences will be lost. You will need to plan how you will learn through your experiences by using a process in which there is an active and interactive process between the learner and the environment (Dewey, 1933). This process is broadly referred to as **experiential learning**.

There are many experiential learning cycles and theories that you may have already heard about in terms of nursing education. It is simply not possible to look at each of these different theories within this book, quite apart from the fact that it is not necessary. The main point is that a learning cycle provides a purposeful and realistic way to learn in, through and during the experiences you will encounter on practice placement. As an added bonus, it is quite simple to learn how to self-regulate your learning experiences by using a learning cycle. However, for the purposes of developing your own self-regulatory skills for learning through clinical experiences, we are going to focus on just one experiential learning approach.

Kolb's experiential learning cycle

Kolb's (1984) process of experiential learning is an easy way for you to start planning how to learn in, through and during an experience. Kolb's model of experiential learning is best described as a four-stage cycle of different

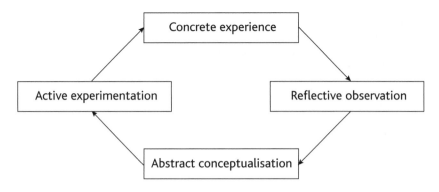

Figure 7.1: Kolb's experiential learning cycle.
Source: Adapted from Kolb (1984, p42).

learning modes (ibid.). Figure 7.1 shows each stage of the cycle clearly. A great feature of the experiential cycle is that each stage – concrete experience, reflective observation, abstract conceptualisation and active experimentation (ibid.) – represents a different aspect of what you might learn during a learning experience.

Concrete experience

You may find that your learning experiences often begin at the concrete experience stage of the learning cycle. This essentially happens because a concrete experience is where you have the opportunity to do something (Dennison and Kirk, 1990). The great part about clinical practice is that you don't have to conjure up your concrete experiences; they occur constantly and you will have no trouble in finding them. Have a look back at Activity 7.1 on page 73. Every single predictable and unpredictable experience that you listed could be classed as a concrete experience.

You will only learn something at this stage, however, if you make links between the experience itself and your learning outcomes (Cantor, 1995). If you have prepared for your placement thoroughly, you should have a very clear understanding of the types of concrete experiences you will need to have during your placement in order to meet learning outcomes. When these events do arise during your placement, you will be able to identify them straightaway and latch on to them as learning opportunities.

In order to learn during a concrete experience, you will also need to reflect on the experience while it is taking place. You will have already been introduced to reflection as a process of deep thought that includes looking back at the situation being pondered upon and projecting forward to the future (Carroll et al., 2001). Jarvis (1992) argues that reflective practice is more than just thoughtful practice; it is the process of turning thoughtful practice into a potential learning situation. Schon (1983) terms this type of reflection as 'reflection-in-action'. It is ideally suited to being utilised within a concrete experience as it involves looking at past experiences, individual values, opinions and expectations in order to handle a current situation; in other words, 'thinking on your feet' (Pattison et al., 2000). If you fail to reflect during a concrete learning experience, it will be very difficult to move into the next stage of the learning cycle, and the value of the experience will be lost.

CASE STUDY 7.2

Ann's placement gets off to a great start and she is enjoying all the different learning experiences available. During her first week she identifies activities that will provide her with opportunities to meet her learning outcomes. Every Wednesday the morning clinic is set aside for adolescents who are undergoing chemotherapy. She decides to use the activities that take place during this clinic to focus on learning outcome number 7 (see Case study 7.1), as a range of therapeutic approaches is used to care for the patients. During one of these clinics Ann has the opportunity to care for Carlos, a 14-year-old boy who is nearing the end of his treatment programme. Carlos is experiencing ongoing nausea as a result of his chemotherapy and is distressed about losing his hair.

Ann listens as her mentor Fiona gives him advice about anti-emetics, explaining how the medications work and the best time to take them. Fiona takes her time with Carlos, giving him the opportunity to express his feelings rather than rushing off to the next patient. When Carlos discloses that his main concern is losing his hair, Fiona talks to him about a support group for teenagers that he could attend. Ann realises that Fiona is gradually building a rapport with Carlos, and that her communication skills are essential to the care she is providing. Ann asks if she can talk to Fiona about Carlos, and they decide to talk in the afternoon as the morning clinic is very busy.

Reflective observation

The next stage in Kolb's experiential learning cycle is a more formalised type of reflection that occurs after the concrete experience event. If a concrete experience can be defined as 'doing', the reflective observation stage is more attune to 'reviewing' (Dennison and Kirk, 1990). In this stage there is a need to reflect on and observe the experiences you have had from many perspectives (Kolb, 1984). In other words, learning occurs through a 'reflection-on-action'. According to Schon (1983) the reflection-on-action that takes place after a concrete experience must be guided so that thinking and practice can be moved forward. Ghaye and Lillyman (2000) contribute to this discussion by suggesting that a reflective conversation should occur following a 'reflection-in-action' event. While this may be perfectly reasonable in theory, the reality of clinical practice means that you may find it very difficult to schedule a reflective conversation with your mentor after every concrete learning experience.

CASE STUDY 7.3

On Wednesday afternoon, Ann and Fiona take their tea break together and talk about the events of the morning. Ann is keen to talk about Carlos and they spend some time reviewing his history, and how his current treatment is resulting in unpleasant side effects. Ann described how she felt when Carlos disclosed his concerns, and Fiona explained how she had decided to spend more time with Carlos as she could sense he was feeling very anxious. Fiona also discusses the need to communicate sensitively with teenagers, who are understandably affected by changes to their body image. They debate the different techniques used in the clinic for treating nausea and hair loss, and Ann is fascinated to learn that aromatherapy is used by some patients to reduce their anxiety. At the end of the tea break Ann realises that there is far more she would like to learn on the subject.

While formal reflection may be difficult due to the busyness of practice areas, in most situations it will be possible to undertake informal reflection following clinical events with your mentor. Ghaye and Lillyman (2008) suggest that this can be achieved by 'reflection-through-practice' and through reflection for the improvement of practice. You will need to self-regulate these reflective sessions, either by prompting your mentor to discuss the experience straightaway or negotiating a convenient time to reflect together. Either way, this will take some motivation on your part, especially as the ability to reflect is the skill in which many adult learners are deficient (Duley, 1980). The main point is that you do undertake some form of reflection on your practice, as Ghaye et al. (1996) believe that, without reflection, it is often impossible to improve practice. Therefore, it can also be argued that, without reflection, it is impossible to learn. In fact, Pattison et al. (2000) go as far as to say that, if we do not embrace reflection, we will never have the opportunity to question the values that underpin our practice and make us the healthcare professionals we claim to be.

REFLECTING DURING PRACTICE PLACEMENT

There are many different ways in which you could use reflection during your practice placement. Take some time now to read through the different types of reflection that may be available to you.

- **Descriptive reflection**   The individual's personal, comprehensive, retrospective account of a situation.
- **Perceptive reflection**   Contains explanations for the feelings of the individual.

- **Receptive reflection** Reflection-on-action. Provides a justification for practice and offers a link between the individual's thinking, feelings and practice, and those of others.

- **Interactive reflection** Reflection shows a link between learning from reflection and future action. A rationale for action is given with the aim of moving practice forward.

- **Critical reflection** Reflection-on-practice. Challenges the status quo and examines the structures that serve to liberate or constrain practice.

Source: Adapted from Pattison et al. (2000, p76).

Abstract conceptualisation

The abstract conceptualisation stage of the experiential learning cycle relates to the thought processes that take place and the subsequent knowledge that you will attain following the concrete experience and your reflective observation. There is no real set formula to what and how you should 'abstractedly conceptualise', as it is your opportunity to make sense of the learning experience following your reflection. It is a bit like a re-evaluation of the experience, in which Boud and Walker (1993) suggest that you can link current experiences with past experiences, integrate the current experience into what you currently know, test for validity and then turn it into your own learning.

It is at this stage of the learning cycle that you may be able to identify your specific strengths and weaknesses, or gaps in your knowledge that need to be addressed. In fact, reflective observation and abstract conceptualisation tend to merge naturally into each other, as it is almost impossible to pinpoint when reflection becomes new insight and vice versa. Pattison et al. (2000) suggest that it is this continuum of reflective practices that distinguishes a nurse from a technician. Yet the main point is that learning takes place as a result of abstract conceptualisation because you are able to create concepts that integrate your observations into logically sound theories (Kolb, 1984). It is this movement through the learning cycle that allows for learning in, through and during experiences.

CASE STUDY 7.4

After talking with Fiona, Ann realises that she would like to learn more about the support and advice available for adolescents with cancer. Over the course of the next week, she makes a point of attending an MDT meeting and has the opportunity of observing a teenage support group meeting where relaxation techniques, including aromatherapy and massage, are available. She also realises that her knowledge of chemotherapy and anti-emetic medications is limited and she uses some placement time to study the literature and increase her knowledge of the medications.

Active experimentation

The last stage of Kolb's experiential learning cycle is defined as active experimentation and, as the term suggests, this part of the cycle is event orientated. In fact, on the surface it is very similar to the concrete experience stage as there is an activity going on here – something is happening. However, active experimentation is not just concerned with the event or experience itself. It is the application stage of the cycle where the emphasis is on practical applications as opposed to reflective understanding; there is a pragmatic concern with what works, on influencing people and changing situations (Kolb, 1984). In other words, active experimentation is all about applying knowledge. You experience an event, you think about it, you make sense of what happened and then you adjust your practices as a result of what you have learned. Dennison and Kirk (1990) propose that, if the learning cycle up to this point has been successful, you will have the capacity and understanding to act differently.

It is important to note that, while active experimentation is the last stage of the learning cycle, it provides the opportunity for a new beginning rather than an end. By moving through a complete learning cycle you will be capable of behaving in a way that you would not have known previously when you are next confronted with a new situation (Dennison and Kirk, 1990). Your experiences of moving through one cycle will naturally open up opportunities to engage with new concrete experiences that will start another cycle all over again. Perhaps this is best summed up by Kolb (1984) in his assertion that we can all learn from our experiences and the results of this learning will pull us through.

CASE STUDY 7.5

The following Wednesday, Carlos returns to the day-care clinic. Ann works with Fiona to set up his chemotherapy and is pleased to find that she now has a better understanding of why the chemotherapy must be given in a certain order. Carlos mentions that his nausea has been reduced and his appetite has improved. Ann talks to him about his new chemotherapy regime and, as his treatment progresses through the morning, she is able to answer most of his questions. Ann's experience with Carlos has made her recognise the importance of establishing trust, being sensitive to the needs of her patients and, most importantly, treating each patient as an individual. Now that she has learned some of these skills, she decides to get more involved in support groups for patients in the day-care clinic. She discusses her options with Fiona and arranges to shadow one of the nurse specialists the next day.

Ann continues to seek out and expand her learning experiences for the remaining weeks of her clinical placement. She achieves all outcomes and takes away with her an expanse of new knowledge, skills and professionalism that she can transfer into her future learning experiences.

Your style of learning

Not only does Kolb's experiential learning cycle (Kolb, 1984) provide a comprehensive plan for learning, it also allows you to blend your preferred learning style into the learning cycle. You should already have a clear understanding of your preferred learning style, and also the style of learning that is least like you. We dealt with this in Chapter 4. Remember that you will need to use facets of all learning styles in order to make the most of your learning opportunities and also develop competence. Kolb's learning cycle makes this possible, as each stage of the learning cycle matches one type of learning style. In Figure 7.2, it should be clear that each part of the learning cycle supports a different type of learning style.

This means that every learning activity that you engage with in practice will have at least one aspect that matches your own preferred learning style. Therefore, if you are a theorist you may choose to begin your learning cycle at the abstract conceptualisation stage; likewise, an activist may choose to begin their learning at the concrete experience stage. It is important to remember that there is no right or wrong way to begin a learning cycle; the most important thing is that you do move sequentially through each stage of the cycle to ensure that you have made the most of each opportunity. This will give you a chance to practise and develop the learning style that you least prefer and, in so doing, move towards developing your nursing competence.

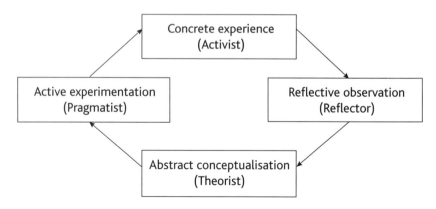

Figure 7.2: Kolb's experiential learning cycle and learning style.
Source: Adapted from Kolb (1984, p42) and Honey and Mumford (1992, p7).

CHAPTER SUMMARY

We all have the potential to learn in, through and during experiences. However, learning doesn't just happen by itself. In order to learn from your clinical experience you will first need to want to learn, and then deliberately set out to learn. Kolb's experiential learning cycle provides an opportunity to completely engage with a learning experience while on clinical placement. Not only will learning become more enjoyable, but your experiences and subsequent reflections will open up a world of future learning opportunities that will stimulate further learning. The rewards will be immediate, and the effort you put into your learning will be paid back to you – with interest.

KNOWLEDGE REVIEW

Having completed the chapter, how would you now rate your knowledge of the following topics?

	Good	Adequate	Poor
1. The link between self-regulated learning and learning through experience.			
2. How to apply the principles of a learning cycle, in order to plan your placement learning experiences.			
3. How you can use reflection to learn from placement experiences.			

Where you're not confident in your knowledge of a topic, what will you do next?

Further reading

Dennison, B and Kirk, R (1990) *Do, Review, Learn, Apply: A simple guide to experiential learning.* Oxford: Blackwell Education.
This book provides an easy-to-read overview of experiential learning, with simple descriptions of theory and practical examples and case studies.

Useful websites

www.learningandteaching.info/learning/experience.htm This website provides a great overview of the experiential learning model and its relationship to learning styles.
www.businessballs.com/kolblearningstyles.htm A detailed look at Kolb's experiential learning cycle with suggestions on how to incorporate learning styles into a learning sequence.

CHAPTER AIMS

The aim of this chapter is to assist you with understanding the role of feedback in relation to your learning experience and assessment of competence.

After reading this chapter you will be able to:

- identify the key aspects of verbal and written feedback;
- understand the relevance of feedback in facilitating learning;
- appreciate the role of the mentor in delivering feedback.

Introduction: feedback

It is quite common for students on clinical placement to be desperate to receive feedback from their mentor. Understandably, you will want to be given regular updates about your performance. As you are likely to be preoccupied with receiving a good report (Cahill, 1996), feedback can provide reassurance on your progress and an opportunity to improve if there are any problems. Ideally, you will want timely, balanced and respectful feedback (Kelly, 2007). To a certain extent you are reliant on your mentor to give feedback on your clinical practice, so that you can improve your level of performance (Glover, 2000).

In this chapter we will be discussing how feedback is a vital aspect of your learning experience. We will start by looking at some common problems with feedback and the relationship between feedback and assessment, and you will also gain an insight into your mentor's role regarding feedback. The chapter will then explore why feedback is so important in helping you become a self-regulated learner. There will be an opportunity to reflect on your previous experiences in receiving feedback, and also to review when you should get feedback and the different types you can expect to receive. We will also look at the importance of understanding your own reactions to feedback in order to be able to learn from it. In addition, we will discuss how formal and informal feedback can be incorporated into a learning cycle. The chapter will conclude by looking at issues related to the documentation of feedback.

Problems with feedback

In the past, students have reported numerous problems with the feedback they receive from mentors. It is often given too late, is destructive rather than constructive, is personal in nature and fails to concentrate on skill (Cahill, 1996). When feedback fails to concentrate on skill development and enhanced clinical performance, it is typical for a student's reaction to become negative (Clynes and Raftery, 2008). For this reason, Dohrenwend (2002) points out that feedback should be an evaluation of performance, not an evaluation of character. It is clear, therefore, that mentors have a responsibility for delivering accurate and fair feedback. However, before you are tempted to become too judgemental and critical of mentors, it is worth looking at feedback from their perspective.

Assessment and feedback

An essential part of your assessment while on clinical placement requires your mentor to provide you with feedback. Your assessment will be undertaken using an assessment tool, with the aim being for your mentor to provide an accurate and objective assessment of your competence (Chambers, 1998; Watson et al., 2002). While assessment documents vary according to your university, they invariably contain the same fundamental elements. The provision of feedback to students is one of these elements. In a study conducted by Gray and Smith (2000), students identified the provision of feedback as an attribute of a 'good' mentor. Yet, despite ample evidence to suggest the value and necessity of feedback within the mentoring role, there is also evidence to suggest that some mentors may be either failing to deliver feedback, or failing in the delivery of feedback. This is quite obviously of some concern, given that the provision of effective feedback is viewed as an essential element within the assessment process (RCN, 2005).

Failing to give feedback

For many mentors, giving feedback to students is one of the biggest challenges and most difficult aspects of their role. Many mentors find that the delivery of feedback is inhibited by the pressures of clinical supervision, inadequate staffing levels, heavy workloads and lack of continuity of support (Aston and Molassiotis, 2003). There is a multitude of reasons why mentors fail to deliver feedback, the most common being:

- time restraints;
- competing clinical pressures;
- sick leave;
- night duty;
- annual leave.

Of course, the irony is that the periods of intense clinical activity tend to be the moments when you will require maximum support and feedback (Clynes and Raftery, 2008). If a mentor fails to give feedback, this is a problem, as providing time for reflection, feedback, monitoring and documenting of a student's progress are key responsibilities of a mentor (RCN, 2007).

Student reactions to feedback

It is not uncommon for highly skilled and experienced mentors to experience fear at the thought of giving a student feedback regarding their performance. In fact, it is well known that some mentors have been so reluctant to give feedback to students that they have avoided doing it at all. Clynes and Raftery (2008) highlight that, despite careful preparation, some mentors may choose to delay or avoid evaluation meetings with students for fear of a negative response or overreaction to criticism.

CASE STUDY 8.1

It is the third week of Mary's clinical placement and she is being supervised by her mentor, Denis, on a drug round. Denis has noticed on previous occasions that Mary struggles with drug calculations, and frequently forgets the formulas she should be using. He has pointed this out to her and has even offered to help with practising calculations on quiet shifts. Once again, during the drug round Mary struggles with her calculations and Denis decides to provide some feedback once the drug round is over. He is concerned that, if Mary does not show significant improvement, she will not meet a competent level. Mary reacts very badly to the feedback she receives from Denis. She accuses him of picking on her, as he has not spoken to other students about their drug calculations. She tells Denis that he puts too much pressure on her, and if he were not there she is sure she would be able to perform calculations. She decides that Denis has it in for her and requests a new mentor.

The truth of the matter is that some students may not always accept a mentor's feedback, even if it is accurate, as they have a very poor understanding of their own level of performance. In Case study 8.1, if Mary does not believe that she has any shortcomings, she may well feel that her mentor is being unfair. This means that, as a student, you must be prepared to receive all feedback, and not just the feedback that you wish to hear. It is not easy for your mentor to provide feedback, and almost impossible if you react badly to it.

The feedback you receive from a mentor is fundamentally based on their opinion. As a result, your feedback will be largely determined by:

- *what your mentor sees;*
- *how significant your mentor thinks it is;*
- *how your mentor interprets what they have seen;*
- *whether what your mentor sees may contribute to your current or future actions.*

(Eraut, 2006, p111)

Learning from feedback

The ability to learn and make use of the feedback you receive on placement is once again related to your self-regulatory skills in relation to your learning. Not only are you responsible for your learning, but you also have a responsibility to respond appropriately to the feedback you are given regarding your performance. We all want to hear the best about ourselves and, if feedback does not do this, there is a natural tendency to feel that it is inaccurate. This is not to say that you must believe automatically everything you are told, as mentors do not always get it right. However, you will need the skills to take on board the feedback you are given and evaluate your own performance objectively. Being able to self-assess your own performance is an advanced skill, but it is not impossible to learn and will only serve to enhance your own learning.

Johari window

A Johari window exercise (see Activity 8.1) is a great way to understand that there is more to you than the way you perceive or understand things. Each of the four windows represents an aspect of you – your personality – that is relevant to the way you view the world and others view you. It is a way of accepting who you are.

- The first window, 'Known by self/Known by others', represents facts that you know and others equally know about you. For example, your favourite colour is purple, and all your friends know that your favourite colour is purple.

- The second window, 'Unknown by self/Known by others', represents things that you may not know about yourself, but that others know about you. For example, you may not realise that you frown when you talk, but everyone who speaks to you recognises this.

- The third window, 'Known by self/Unknown by others', represents things that you know about yourself, but others don't know about you. For example, your favourite food is lamb hotpot, but only you know this.

- The fourth window, 'Unknown by self/Unknown by others', represents what you don't yet know about yourself, and others don't know about you either. These are often parts of your character that are yet to be discovered, for example how you might react if you won the lottery. Unless you actually win the lottery, no one, including yourself, will ever know.

ACTIVITY 8.1

Have a go at filling out the box yourself, and then ask others to contribute as well. You may get quite a surprise by what others have observed about you, but not shared with you.

1. Known by self/Known by others	2. Unknown by self/Known by others
3. Known by self/Unknown by others	4. Unknown by self/Unknown by others

Source: Adapted from Dennison and Kirk (1990, p29).

You may wonder what relevance the Johari window has to feedback on clinical practice. The simple answer is that, when you understand the principles of a Johari window, it becomes clear that you are not always the best judge of yourself. Some things that take place in practice will be clear and straightforward, and both you and your mentor may agree on some of your strengths and weaknesses (window 1). However, there will be things that your mentor will pick up about your performance in practice that you are unaware of (window 2). There will be reasons for why you respond to certain situations in practice that only you understand (window 3). Finally, you will be exposed to new situations in practice that require you to take part in, or react to, a fresh experience (window 4). In all these instances, your mentor will be able to provide feedback, so you may end up hearing and learning brand new information about yourself that you have never realised. If you are prepared for this, you will stand a great chance of learning and developing from this feedback.

Past experiences of feedback

It may be that you have already had experiences of receiving feedback from a mentor. Some of those experiences may have been positive, and some may have been unsatisfactory. It is worth reflecting on previous experiences you may have in receiving feedback, as this may highlight any issues you have in relation to asking for or receiving feedback.

ACTIVITY 8.2

Use the chart below to identify the factors that contributed to both the positive and negative feedback experiences you have had in the past. If you can relate your experiences to previous practice placements this would be useful; however, you can also look at past work-related performance reviews.

My feedback experience was positive because . . .

My feedback experience was negative because . . .

There will be key areas of each feedback situation that were fundamental to the eventual result. It may be that the negative feedback experience could have been avoided if you had been equipped with additional knowledge and skill in relation to how you could have responded to feedback at the time of the event. Alternatively, Clynes and Raftery (2008) have identified that the preparation of mentors in delivering feedback to students is paramount. If your mentor is lacking the confidence and skill to give fair and accurate feedback, you may have a less than positive experience. Young (2000) cites feedback as a delicate balancing act between fair assessment and protecting vulnerable students. While students value feedback from mentors (Kelly, 2007), mentors are not always prepared for the delivery of feedback (Eraut, 2006). This means that you must not only be prepared for feedback, but also ensure that you are open to receiving feedback by encouraging mentors to do this throughout your placement.

When should I receive feedback?

We have already established that students expect feedback. You will want to hear comments from your mentor on how you are performing. Keeping this in mind, you should be open to receiving feedback from the very beginning of your placement. While the literature supports that providing feedback to nursing students is imperative (Eaton, 1995), just how and when to do this remains a matter for conjecture. Mentors are advised by the NMC that they essentially have a responsibility to provide students with feedback as often as it is needed to guide performance. As discussed in Chapter 3, *The Standards to Support Learning and Assessment in Practice* (NMC, 2008) reiterate that this is especially important within the context of the sign-off mentor role.

> *Sign-off mentors will require allocated time to ensure that students have effective feedback on their performance so that the ultimate decision on their proficiency is not unexpected. The time allocated may need to be greater earlier in the placement and reduced as they become more confident and competent.*

(NMC, 2008, p33)

Remember that feedback is an essential aspect of your formative assessment, and it can help you to rate your clinical performance more realistically (Glover, 2000). If you are not reaching a competent standard, feedback should be more frequent to provide opportunities to develop and improve. However, your mentor does need to ensure that they are not overdoing your feedback, as you may feel threatened by this. It is essential, therefore, that you have a clear understanding of the two different types of feedback that you may encounter throughout your placement in order to prepare for what to do in these situations.

Keeping it casual

Informal feedback occurs randomly throughout a clinical placement and is usually given by your mentor in response to a specific event. It can happen at any time and is generally unplanned. It may take place on the spot or as an informal conversation some time later (Eraut, 2006). In general, the earlier that informal feedback becomes routine between a mentor and student during a placement, the better. Both you and your mentor will benefit from establishing frequent and spontaneous lines of communication. It is well established that insufficient feedback can impact negatively on your learning experience. Some students have described that the lack of openness of their mentors' feedback increased their anxiety and insecurity during clinical placement (Cahill, 1996). However, if feedback is regularly given on the spot, it can be supportive and constructive and can provide opportunities for reflection (Eraut, 2006).

Mentors also benefit from providing students with regular feedback, as they also gain confidence in discussing your progress. However, you must be very careful not to request continual feedback from your mentor, and it is more than reasonable for them to put some limitations on the amount of feedback you receive. If you do want to receive frequent feedback, you may choose to plan ahead with your mentor for specific time periods where this may be possible. It is also a good idea to put a defined time limit on the discussion (Atkins and Williams, 1995), so that no one becomes frustrated.

Keep in mind that either you or your mentor can instigate feedback and you do not have to wait for your mentor to provide it; in fact, it is in your best interest to request it. Your mentor may volunteer feedback, but if they don't, then ask for it.

Black tie optional

Formal feedback is a planned event and it will normally take place at predetermined stages of the clinical placement, namely the initial interview, midpoint review and end assessment. It should be structured and ideally be conducted in a quiet area away from the general environment of clinical work. Dohrenwend (2002) concludes that privacy and allowing adequate time for what is said to be digested is vital when giving feedback. It should be noted that your mentor is obliged to provide formative feedback on a regular basis (Eraut, 2006). However, some mentors find it particularly difficult to instigate and deliver feedback in a formal setting, partly due to the strong emotional dimension of the interaction (Eraut, 2006). You may also feel vulnerable when receiving feedback (Dohrenwend, 2002), as this is your mentor's opinion of your performance, and will be directly related to the final decision they make for your placement learning outcomes (Sharples, 2007c). You should be given some time and warning to prepare yourself for the formal feedback event. If you are not given sufficient warning of a formal interview, you may feel quite intimidated and be reluctant to voice your opinions or concerns. A lack of two-way interaction will jeopardise the interaction needed for insight and development (Clynes and Raftery, 2008). To avoid this situation, you should negotiate with your mentor at the start of a placement the dates when formal feedback in the form of midpoint and end interviews is likely to take place. You can then both feel prepared for these meetings as they will become a routine part of your placement.

What feedback should I get?

Regardless of whether you are receiving formal or informal feedback from your mentor, it must always be clear and unambiguous. If you receive too little information, you may be unsure of what is required of you or how this relates to your learning outcomes. On the one hand, when information is withheld, feedback becomes a superficial exercise that lacks the necessary depth to tackle the issues at hand (Dohrenwend, 2002). On the other hand, if feedback includes too much information, you may feel overwhelmed, taking in little of what your mentor has actually said. Clynes and Raftery (2008) comment that feedback should include examples from practice, as well as specific targets and standards. For this reason, Glover (2000) concludes that feedback should be focused on what you can use, rather than the amount your mentor may wish to give.

Lyn is supervising Eunice, who is giving an intramuscular (IM) injection. Eunice calculates the drug dose accurately, and collects the necessary equipment. She then draws up the anti-emetic appropriately and begins to give the injection. However, she forgets to draw back on the syringe and Lyn has to remind her to do it. Eunice continues with the injection, which she performs competently. They leave the patient's bedside and Lyn decides to give Eunice some feedback. However, she feels awkward about doing this as Eunice has not responded well to feedback in the past. She makes a passing comment that Eunice should 'do some more injections while you are here'.

What Lyn really thinks

That is the third time now that she has forgotten to draw back when giving an injection. I don't want to make a big issue of it because it's only her fourth week here, but she's not competent yet. She might think I'm picking on her if I say something. I've told her to practise more, so hopefully she'll remember next time and get better.

What Eunice really thinks

I'm getting really good at injections now. My mentor even wants me to do more. None of the other students has been asked to do more injections, so I must be doing really well. I should be able to get my book signed off next time.

You will not be able to change behaviour if you do not know what needs to be corrected (Dohrenwend, 2002). Therefore, you cannot and must not rely on assumptions or inferences when you are receiving feedback. For this reason it is vital that, once feedback has been delivered, you clarify what has been said by your mentor in order to rectify any misconceptions. You should remember that the feedback you have heard may not always be the same as the feedback given (Eraut, 2006). In fact, Clynes and Raftery (2008) suggest that students should be encouraged to reflect on their mentor's feedback and outline their interpretation of its content.

Constructive feedback

The question of what to discuss and in what way is a constant issue in a feedback situation (Kilbourn, 1990). Within organisational, educational and business domains there has been a great deal of research done into optimum situations and techniques for giving both written and verbal feedback. There is general consensus that constructive feedback is essential and should be frequent (Kilminster et al., 2007), as this will assist students to improve their performance (Sharples, 2007c).

A lack of clarity in feedback can have a detrimental effect on the student/ mentor relationship and can compromise the self-esteem of both. Your mentor must always ensure that the feedback given is constructive, whether it is delivered formally or informally. This means that it should be objective, non-judgemental and based on specific observations, encouraging discussion and allowing for a positive course to be set for the future (Pearce, 2004). If given appropriately, constructive feedback can boost student confidence, motivation and self-esteem (Baard and Neville, 1996). It is not difficult, therefore, to understand the value of constructive feedback, especially as it supports and encourages learning, motivating students to try again, do better or keep up the good work (Steves, 2005). Likewise, mentors also benefit from providing feedback to students through sharing practice and enhancing learning (Allen, 2002).

Incorporating feedback into your learning cycle

The feedback you receive will make a major difference to your learning experience. On-the-spot feedback from your mentor may typically occur during the learning experiences in which you take part, while informal feedback conversations are more likely to occur during periods of reflection and while you are making sense of your learning experiences. In Figure 8.1, you can see how feedback links with Kolb's experiential learning cycle.

It is not difficult, therefore, to see the link between feedback and learning in, through and during practice. As feedback on clinical performance can be a spontaneous part of the working relationship (Eraut, 2006), it will

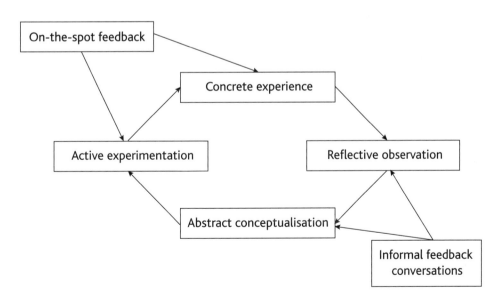

Figure 8.1: Kolb's experiential learning cycle and feedback.
Source: Adapted from Kolb (1984, p42).

naturally open the door to reflection-on-practice (see 'Reflective observation' in Chapter 7, pages 78–9). Pugh (1992) argues that the value of a student undertaking self-reflection of their performance cannot be overestimated, as it will provide valuable insight into the student's perception of their own ability. For this reason, self-reflection should be encouraged in feedback situations. Your self-reflection should also provide opportunities for a clear discussion on strengths and weaknesses with your mentor, and help you to regulate your clinical practice in a realistic way (Glover, 2000). However, without clarity of feedback, the risk is that you may engage in reflective exercises that are not related to the development of clinical competence (Murphy and Atkins, 1994). If you feel that the feedback you are receiving is not constructive, you should address this with your mentor as soon as possible so that learning opportunities are not lost.

Feedback and self-esteem

You may be quite surprised to find that there is a relationship between feedback and the impact it can have on your self-esteem. While honesty from your mentor is important, you may not interpret the feedback as encouraging if you are emotionally reactive or vulnerable due to low self-esteem (London, 1995). This means that the higher your self-esteem, the more positive your attitude towards assessment in general and, more specifically, towards feedback on performance (Young, 2000). Conversely, if you have low self-esteem, you are more likely to have a fear of negative evaluation (Fleming and Courtney, 1984) and, as a consequence, avoid feedback situations as a coping mechanism (Cahill, 1996). Therefore, while students with high self-esteem may view feedback as an opportunity to improve, those with low self-esteem may adopt a defeatist mentality and perhaps even consider leaving the course (Young, 2000). It is not surprising, therefore, that mentors may also be reluctant to engage in feedback with students because they are uncomfortable in giving what may be interpreted as 'bad news' (Steves, 2005). While it may be obvious that students should be provided with feedback couched in positive terms in order to maintain or improve self-esteem, this does create some difficulty when feedback is required to point out errors or poor performance (Begley and White, 2003).

In earlier chapters we dealt with previous experiences of education as a root cause of negative attitudes and poor self-esteem, especially in your ability to learn. Quite understandably, if you have been exposed to unhappy learning experiences in your past, this baggage will affect your self-esteem. In particular, previous negative experiences may result in you reacting negatively to feedback, as it may be difficult to cast aside past experiences. It is crucially important, therefore, that you ask for feedback that is highly specific (Wiggins, 1998) and related to an evaluation of your behaviour and work performance, so that you do not misinterpret it as an evaluation of your character (Russell, 1994).

CASE STUDY 8.3

A student speaks about her experience of receiving feedback on a placement:

In my first year of training I did this placement in this little community hospital and everyone was really friendly and got on well and at first I thought it was a really great placement. In my second week I was really shocked when my mentor called me aside to say that all the nurses had noticed problems with my documenting in patient charts. I took it really badly and ended up in tears. I couldn't understand why I was being singled out, especially as I was only in first year and they were expecting me to be perfect. I was really angry and I told her I didn't think it was fair that the nurses were all talking about me. She was really quiet for a while and I thought, 'That's got her, she can't defend that one.' She just looked at me and said, 'Would you prefer I said nothing and let you keep making the same mistakes?' I thought about that for ages afterwards, and I realise that she was right; she was only trying to help. I'm in third year now and almost ready to qualify. My current mentor is really impressed with my record keeping and soon I'll be signed off as competent. I might not have made it this far if that mentor in my first year had not been so honest.

There is always a tendency for students with low self-esteem to take any comment as an indictment of themselves (Young, 2000), and if you have had previous negative experiences this can be exacerbated. There is nothing wrong with explaining your feelings about feedback to your mentor, and encouraging them to provide feedback that is specific, focused and emotionally sensitive (Eraut, 2006). If this is taken into consideration, you should be able to view feedback as help and advice, rather than a personal attack.

Documenting feedback

The one area in which you may really struggle is the formal documentation of feedback in your assessment documents. This may be because you may not view feedback positively as a direction for change and instead may interpret it as a definitive judgement on ability (Young, 2000). However, without a written record of an event, there is no evidence to support what has been done or said. *The Standards to Support Learning and Assessment in Practice* (NMC, 2008) conclusively demonstrate the position of the NMC in relation to written feedback:

The NMC considers it important that mentors have an audit trail to support their decisions. Throughout a placement where a critical decision on progress is to be made the mentor should ensure that regular feedback is given to the student and that records are kept of guidance given.

(p33)

You must understand that, by recording feedback in your assessment document, your mentor is fulfilling a professional obligation. They are accountable and responsible to the NMC for the assessment decision they make about you (NMC, 2008). This means that the documentation they write must be an accurate record of events. Moreover, the NMC considers documentation to be a vital aspect of the assessment process, as it provides an 'audit trail' to support the decision to pass or fail a student (ibid.). Mentors have no choice; they are professionally obligated to document the feedback they give to you, as this will provide evidence to support the assessment process and their assessment decision (Sharples, 2007c).

What should my mentor write?

The record of feedback that the mentor writes in your assessment document needs to be both fair and accurate. Written feedback should be dated and signed by you and your mentor, as it often forms the basis of a learning contract or action plan. You should expect the verbal and written feedback you are given to be consistent (Sharples, 2007c), as it should provide an opportunity for setting specific standards and targets (Wiggins, 1998). You can also use the documentation of feedback to discuss your learning needs with other nurses and mentors in your clinical area and lecturers from your university.

Where should my mentor write?

Written feedback should be recorded in the assessment document that the university has provided for you. There will generally be a section provided within the document for mentors to write their feedback. This will probably be highlighted as initial, midpoint and end interviews. However, additional information is always welcomed by the universities and it is worth finding out where in the assessment document you should advise your mentor to write extra feedback. It may be in the form of an action plan, Ongoing Achievement Record or general report section. Your mentor will need to write enough for any concerns or assessment decisions to be explained and for you to be aware of what is required of you in order to improve.

CHAPTER SUMMARY

The feedback you receive from your mentor while you are on clinical placement is an essential part of your overall learning experience. This is because feedback provides your mentor with the opportunity of giving you their opinion on your performance. Some mentors struggle with providing feedback, so establishing clear guidelines for how and when feedback will be facilitated is a key aspect of your placement experience. As feedback is based on your mentor's judgement of your competence, it should always be related to the learning outcomes you are trying to achieve. Mentors are professionally obligated to provide students with fair and timely feedback. As we have discovered, it can be particularly challenging to receive feedback if you have low self-esteem, as you are at risk of taking what is said personally. Ideally, feedback should be well timed, well targeted and well said in order to direct growth, motivate and contribute to your learning experience.

KNOWLEDGE REVIEW

Having completed the chapter, how would you now rate your knowledge of the following topics?

	Good	Adequate	Poor
1. The key aspects of verbal and written feedback.			
2. The relevance of the feedback in relation to your learning.			
3. The role and responsibility of the mentor in delivering feedback.			

Where you're not confident in your knowledge of a topic, what will you do next?

Further reading

Eraut, M (2006) Editorial. *Learning in Health and Social Care*, 5(3): 111–18.
This is an easy-to-read article that provides additional insight into the role of feedback and improving work-based performance. Varying types of feedback strategies and tips for constructive communication are discussed.

Useful website

www.businessballs.com/johariwindowmodel.htm This website explores the Johari window in some depth, explaining the variations of each window and how feedback can be used to gain insight and open learning experiences.

9. Learning to learn in practice

CHAPTER AIMS

The aim of this chapter is to identify the role that motivation plays in your practice learning experience, and the potential obstacles to learning that you may encounter.

After reading this chapter you will be able to:

- identify various factors that affect motivation;

- appreciate the difference between intrinsic and extrinsic motivation;

- understand common threats to motivation within clinical practice;

- identify a number of strategies you can use for getting and staying motivated to learn in practice.

Introduction: motivation to learn

Throughout all your placement experiences, there will be times when you encounter a variety of issues, problems and obstacles that, if not overcome, will affect the quality of your learning experience. In some cases, the obstacle may be a general lack of motivation. In other circumstances, issues and problems are encountered that will impact on your motivation.

The first step is to recognise that it is entirely normal to face challenges to your learning while you are in practice. This is not personal to you; the fact is that we do not live in a perfect world and clinical practice, like all aspects of life, is not perfect. The second step is to acknowledge that, in most cases, you can do quite a lot to overcome these problems when they occur. Of course, in order to do this you will need to recognise the nature of these potential obstacles, and then understand what you can do to either prevent or overcome them. Like all problems, the earlier you address them, the smaller they will be. Therefore, while challenges to your learning are almost impossible to avoid, the good news is that, by facing these issues head-on, you can either avoid these pitfalls altogether, or reduce their impact on your learning experience if and when they occur.

Most student nurses at some point in their training are affected by a reduction in, or complete loss of, motivation. In this chapter we will identify what motivation is and the differences between intrinsic and extrinsic motivation. There will be a focus on the factors that can have a detrimental effect on motivation, including:

- fatigue, tiredness and sleep deprivation due to shift work;
- juggling home and work commitments with clinical placement;
- personality clashes with mentors;
- challenges in learning with a disability.

As each of these issues will affect your ability to learn, we will discuss how you might reduce the stress and anxiety they may induce.

Let's get motivated

Motivation is one of those strange things that, while you cannot actually touch it, feel it, taste it or see it, it really does exist and actually will have one of the biggest roles to play in your learning experience. In fact, you will very often rely heavily on motivation in order to learn – so much so that, without motivation, learning will be almost impossible. The paradox is that, while motivation is essential for learning, you cannot buy motivation, nor can you borrow someone else's. Either you have it or you don't, and someone else telling you to get motivated will have little influence at all.

What is motivation?

Before we go any further, it is important to establish exactly what motivation is in order to understand where it comes from and, more importantly, where it goes when it seems to just disappear.

ACTIVITY 9.1

No doubt you have had times in your life when, one day, you felt very motivated towards doing or achieving something, but the next day the feeling just seems to have vanished. It is worth stopping here and reflecting on this experience and it may help to make some brief notes.

- What were the circumstances of this event?
- Why do you think you felt motivated?
- How long did the motivation last?
- When did your motivation disappear?
- Why do you think you lost motivation?

The frustrating thing about losing motivation is that it is not like losing a set of keys; you can't just hunt around looking for places you might have left it. This does not mean that, if you lose motivation, it can't be found again; it simply means that motivation is not a tangible object that can be physically picked up or put down. In its simplest form, **motivation** may be defined as the forces or processes that cause individuals to act in a specific way (Maitland, 1995). However, motivation as a theory and as a method of explaining human behaviour cannot be limited to or explained through just one definition. The problem, of course, as Vernon (1969) explains, is that motivation is such an internal experience that it remains difficult to classify, define or interpret. This is mainly due to the fact that humans do not always fit neatly into precise scientific boxes. Despite these difficulties, many notable theorists have attempted to, and indeed continue to, interpret and promote our understanding of human motivation.

Maslow's hierarchy of needs

One such theorist was Abraham Maslow, a behavioural scientist who developed a theory about the rank and satisfaction of various human needs. This is widely referred to today as **Maslow's hierarchy of needs**. Maslow (1943) based his motivational theory on the concept that the integrated wholeness of the organism must be one of the foundation stones of human motivation. In other words, your motivation is directly related to who you are, your personality and what makes you 'tick'. His theory of motivation proposed that all individuals have a set hierarchy of needs that they have a desire to satisfy (Maitland, 1995). In addition, Maslow (1943) argued that humans need to arrange themselves in hierarchies, where the appearance of one need rests on the prior satisfaction of others. The order of these needs is represented in Figure 9.1.

It is quite easy to see that, in order of needs, motivation begins with the satisfaction of physiological needs and progresses in turn through needs related

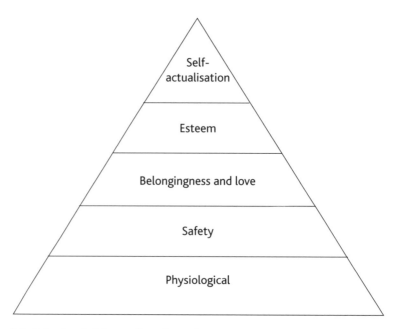

Figure 9.1: Maslow's hierarchy of needs.
Source: Adapted from Maslow (1987, pp15–22).

to safety, belongingness and love, esteem and self-actualisation (Maslow, 1987). In its simplest form, Maitland (1995) suggests that Maslow's motivational theory allows individuals to move up through the various levels of the hierarchical pyramid once these classified needs are developed, satisfied and fulfilled at each level.

Learning and motivation

It is worth pointing out here that, by undertaking your nursing training, you are striving for the top two levels of the pyramid. The act of learning, increasing your knowledge, is associated with a need for esteem and self-actualisation. On the one hand, this is great news and you should rightly be proud of yourself for wanting to attain this level. However, on the other hand, it is not difficult to see that the higher up the pyramid you go, the greater risk there is that something at a lower stage may impact on your higher-order motivation. In fact, many student nurses feel that Murphy's Law – 'If it can go wrong, it will go wrong' – was written especially for them.

ACTIVITY 9.2

Each stage of Maslow's hierarchy of needs represents a range of different needs. The premise is that we need to feel fulfilled at each stage before the next stage of the motivational pyramid can be reached. Have a look at the examples below to see the types of needs that are represented at each stage.

Self-actualisation	Confidence, achievement, personal growth, fulfilment
Esteem	Recognition, reputation, dignity, status
Belongingness and love	Family, friends, partner, children
Safety	Job security, shelter, health
Physiological	Food, water, air, warmth, sleep

Take some time to refer back to the notes you made in Activity 9.1. Try to identify where you were on the motivational pyramid when you felt motivated. What 'need' were you satisfying while you were at this level? Now look at the categories below this level. Can you identify a change in your circumstances that may have influenced your motivation? Perhaps you were motivated to improve an aspect of your esteem when something happened to change your feeling of safety. If this was the case, you would have quickly lost motivation for improving your esteem and focused on re-establishing your safety.

It is quite easy to see how physiological needs are the priority in the motivational pyramid. Our most basic needs in life are those that keep us alive and, if these are at risk, it is not difficult to understand that there would be little motivation to move on to the next stage of the pyramid. This isn't to say that all examples of needs must be met, but we must feel secure and happy at each level before we can move on. In fact, pivotal to Maslow's motivational theory is his belief that any motivated behaviour is a channel through which many basic needs may simultaneously be expressed or satisfied (Maslow, 1943). In other words, your motivation to do or not do something is rarely down to just one factor. A whole range of influences will contribute to your overall motivation, and these can occur at any stage of the motivational pyramid. This also means that your motivation will be influenced by a combination of needs that contribute to your personality.

SCENARIO

Sarah works for a multinational insurance firm and has spent many years building up her reputation and progressing within the organisation. Her dream is to become one day the managing director of the company and she has spent her entire career working towards this ultimate goal. One day, she is informed that a new post is being developed and she spends days preparing for the interview, as this will be one more stepping stone towards her ultimate goal. On the day of the interview her partner becomes very ill and is rushed to hospital. Within seconds, all Sarah's motivation for the new job and interview disappears. Her priority changes instantly, from promoting her own need for esteem to protecting her need for belongingness and love. It is only once she is assured that her partner will make a full recovery that she can once again concentrate on, and motivate herself towards, personal ambitions.

Like all skills, developing ways to motivate yourself for learning will require some practice. Your nursing course should have already provided you with some skills for planning your practice learning, for example interpersonal, communication, decision-making, negotiation and problem-solving skills. These are all assets that you can use in order to motivate yourself when the placement commences. However, as Sharples et al. (2007) recognise, it is naive to assume that all nursing students entering clinical placement will have the knowledge, skills and attitude to be successful. It may well be that motivation is missing. If you are lacking motivation, you must do something to rectify this.

Intrinsic and extrinsic motivation

We have already established that motivation is strongly related to events that happen around you and also your personality. Obviously, there will be events that take place outside your control that will ultimately affect your motivation.

However, in some instances you can change or predict the clinical placement events that may affect your motivation and, in doing so, protect the quality of your learning experience. It is important to recognise, however, that while a loss of motivation during a clinical placement will rarely mean the end of a placement, it will usually signify a loss of interest in learning during the placement. If you happen to be on clinical placement with no interest in learning, there is little point being there.

The ball is in your court

While it is not difficult to understand that seizing learning opportunities will be important to your placement experience, having the motivation to do this is an entirely different matter. The reason for this may be related to the origin of your motivation. Is your motivation intrinsic or extrinsic? **Intrinsic motivation** is generally considered to be associated with achieving a goal or performing a task for its own sake. On the other hand, **extrinsic motivation** stems from a desire for reward (Benabou and Tirole, 2003). In most cases you will find that both types of motivation will contribute to your overall motivation on clinical placement and there is no problem with this. However, you will run into difficulties if you depend entirely on extrinsic motivational forces, as these can fluctuate and dissipate very quickly. If you rely on being rewarded as a means of generating your motivation, what will happen if the rewards stop or are not as frequent as you would like? Obviously, your motivation will also suffer. It may be, then, that your motivation for seeking out and engaging with learning experiences wanes because it is rooted in extrinsic motivational forces rather than grounded in intrinsic aspects of your personality.

A key aspect of maintaining your motivation to learn is through understanding and accepting that your motivation is intrinsic to you. In other words, you will need to accept your own responsibility for learning in, through and during practice (Elcock et al., 2007). In order to fulfil your learning plan, you will need to be motivated enough to negotiate your learning needs (Begley and Brady, 2002). If you are dependent on extrinsic forces for motivation, the likelihood is that you will be unable to shift from task-based activities to a holistic model of learning (Spouse, 2003). If you are not motivated to learn, it is very unlikely that anyone, especially your mentor, will be motivated to stimulate your learning for you.

The implications of these sentiments for your learning in practice are very clear. You can reasonably expect that your nursing course will provide a programme that will guide you in the skills and attributes that you will require for practice learning. However, there is also an equal and incredibly important responsibility for you to seize the opportunities to learn afforded you by your supernumerary status. It is disappointing, therefore, that current research concludes that the supernumerary status of students has failed to make a significant difference to the way many students learn in practice (Elcock et al., 2007). Assuming that you have been provided with the necessary skills for learning in practice, failure to seize opportunities afforded by supernumerary status must be directly related to lack of motivation. The fact is that, if you fail to plan your learning and are not assertive in requesting opportunities to undertake activities, you will miss out on valuable learning experiences (Elcock, 2006).

Here are some examples of different types of motivation that may contribute to your practice experience.

Extrinsic motivation

- Positive feedback from a mentor.
- Passing a practice placement.
- Praise from a patient or client.
- Admiration from family or friends.

Intrinsic motivation

- An overall desire to learn.
- Wanting to increase your own knowledge and skill.
- Learning from your mistakes.
- Developing your professional role.

Can you see the difference between extrinsic and intrinsic motivation? Can you also see that extrinsic motivation tends to be associated with short-term rewards, whereas intrinsic motivation tends to be associated with the bigger picture – perhaps even long-term goals or aspirations? While there is nothing wrong with having extrinsic factors within your motivational drivers, there must also be some element of intrinsic motivation to counterbalance this when extrinsic factors are limited.

ACTIVITY 9.3

Take the time now to make a list of the things that you rely on to motivate you during your clinical placement. You may like to reflect on a previous specific placement experience as a reference point for your ideas. Separate your motivation during this experience into extrinsic and intrinsic factors.

Extrinsic motivation	Intrinsic motivation

Think about the rewards that you may rely on for your extrinsic motivation.

- Do you require these hourly, daily or weekly to sustain motivation?
- What happens if you do not get the rewards you require?
- Do you have intrinsic motivation that you can refer back to and rely on if extrinsic motivation does not take place?

Why do I lose motivation?

The reason that you may lose motivation while on clinical placement will be very personal to you. However, if you do tend to lose motivation, you may find that your core motivational drivers are heavily dependent on extrinsic factors. You will need to develop some intrinsic drivers to cover the periods when extrinsic factors diminish. If you can't think of any intrinsic factors, you may need to think about the fundamental reason that you embarked on a career in nursing in the first place. Did you begin this journey with intrinsic motivation? If so, these initial reasons and feelings should be far more solid and reliable than any extrinsic motivational drivers – and they will need to be. They will need to sustain you through both the good times and the difficult times.

CASE STUDY 9.1

A former student speaks about her motivation to complete her nursing course.

I'm not really sure why I wanted to be a nurse. I guess I just fell into it. There was a lot of pressure from home to do something when I finished college and I had a friend who was doing nursing so I sort of thought, why not? It was ok for a while, but then I had this really difficult placement; I had to travel a long way, I was always tired and I had all this pressure with theory assignments due in. I seriously thought about quitting, I just couldn't see much point in going on. Luckily for me, I came to my senses and realised that it wouldn't always be this bad and if I hung in there it could be a career for life. I'm two years qualified now and I can honestly say that I love my work; not a day goes by when I don't learn something new. I'm even off to work as a nurse in Australia for a year. If I had given up that just wouldn't be possible.

Obstacles to learning

There are several key areas or obstacles that can impact on the learning experience during a clinical placement. In fact, it is often these obstacles that are to blame for a loss or lack of motivation, especially extrinsic motivation. These can range from simple things, such as tiredness and sleep deprivation, to more challenging obstacles, such as personal commitments related to home and family life, financial concerns and personality clashes. In addition, students with disabilities can face particular challenges and may quickly lose motivation if obstacles are not overcome. Therefore, it is important to understand that, until you address your own personal barriers and obstacles to motivation, you will not be able to seize all the learning opportunities available in your supernumerary role.

Motivation and sleep

Sleep is one of our most basic human needs. If we don't get enough sleep, we quickly lose the ability to function as efficiently as we would like. Take another look at Activity 9.2 and see where sleep fits into Maslow's hierarchy of needs. You can see that it forms one of the most basic physiological needs and, without enough sleep, it would be very difficult to motivate yourself further. However, it is also very clear that shift work is notorious for interrupting sleep patterns and contributing to sleep deprivation. Anecdotally, many nurses report that working the night shift and adjusting to sleeping during the day causes the most stress. As a result, many shift workers exist in a constant state of sleep deprivation (Stryjewski and Slonim, 2002). The problem is, of course, that, if you are experiencing sleep deprivation, your motivation to learn will also suffer.

There is a certain irony here, as the NMC has made it quite clear that, in order to develop an understanding of your patients' and clients' experiences of healthcare, you must participate in the full range of 24-hour/7 days a week shifts (NMC, 2004). By default, this means that you will need to undertake shift work as a part of your learning experience, and participate in a combination of early, late and night shifts. While this is primarily designed to give students insight into the needs of their patients over 24 hours of a day, sleep deprivation due to shift work may cause you to lose motivation to learn. Therefore, in order to stay motivated, you will need to 'learn' how to cope with shift work.

TIPS FOR SURVIVING SHIFT WORK

- Avoid caffeinated drinks after midnight. While they may help to keep you awake during the night, they also make it difficult to sleep the next morning.
- Wear sunglasses home from work, even on a cloudy day. The reduced light may help convince your brain that it is night.
- Sleep in a cool room. Body temperature drops at night, so it helps to recreate this coolness when trying to sleep during the day.
- If you like to watch television before bed, record a programme from the night before. It may help to trick your brain into thinking it is night-time.
- Invest in blackout curtains and earplugs. Too much light and noise will stimulate your brain and prevent restful sleep.

Source: Adapted from Sharples and Kelly (2006).

Home and family commitments

There can be no doubt that your home, family and social life will be
impacted by your nurse training, especially during times of clinical
placement. In fact, some students only realise once they arrive on a clinical
placement just how disruptive and challenging this aspect of their training
will be, with family and social life at the mercy of a rolling series of late,
early and weekend shifts (Sharples, 2006). In Chapter 5 we looked at this
particular aspect of your clinical experience in relation to preparation for
placement. However, no matter how prepared you are, the reality is that,
once on placement, your motivation may well suffer if the terms of your
placement are having a negative impact on those you love. Sometimes,
no matter how well planned and thought out, there may be times when this
will happen.

Have another look at Maslow's hierarchy of needs pyramid on page 100 and
where your need to fulfil home and family commitments is placed. You will
see that it fits in with your fundamental need for belongingness and love.
If this is threatened during your clinical experience, the result will be a
loss of, or reduction in, motivation to learn. In these circumstances,
solutions can be quite difficult to find. Ultimately, preparation is vital and,
in this case, being forewarned can result in being forearmed. You will need
to accept that your clinical placements will affect your social and family
life, so you will need to have a plan for how to cope with this before the
placement begins (Sharples, 2006). You may also need to accept that,
where difficulties are outside your control or cannot be resolved, you
may need to take a break in your programme until such time as the issue or
problem has been dealt with. If you are having ongoing problems within your
home and family life that are impacting on your clinical experience, these will
take precedence, and no amount of intrinsic motivation will override these
difficulties.

CASE STUDY 9.2

Wendy has always wanted a career in nursing and decides that, when her youngest
child reaches school age, she will commence her training. She is a single parent and
has made arrangements for her sister to care for her two children during evening,
night and weekend shifts while she is on clinical placement. During her first year of
training this arrangement suits everybody; her children are well cared for by their aunt,
and Wendy can concentrate on her studies. However, in her second year of training the
arrangement falls apart. Wendy's sister becomes ill and can no longer care for the
children. Wendy tries to make alternative arrangements; however, she cannot afford
after-school child care and her children are unhappy being cared for by different
friends every day. As she has no options for night or weekend care, Wendy cannot
commit to the placement rota and is forced to take sick leave on these shifts. The last
thing on Wendy's mind, when she is able to be on placement, is learning from the

experience, as she has lost all motivation. She has no option but to take a break from the programme and she defers for six months. During this time, she is able to care for her sister and she no longer feels stressed as her children are happy. At the end of the six months, Wendy's sister is fully recovered and is able to resume caring for the children. Wendy is able to return to her training at the point she left, fully committed and focused on her learning.

Overcoming personality clashes with mentors

No matter how motivated you are before a clinical placement, this can soon diminish if you have a personality clash with your mentor. Just as there are no perfect mentors, there are no perfect students, and it is a fact of life that, from time to time, personality clashes do occur. This will happen in all aspects of your life, and clinical practice is no different in this respect. Clashes can occur for any number of reasons and it would be rare to find that there is not some level of fault on both sides. This is not to say that nothing can be done to reduce or eradicate personality clashes, as there is a range of solutions to these types of problems. However, it does need to be understood that personality clashes are almost impossible to prevent, and at some point you will no doubt have a clash of personalities with a mentor.

It also needs to be said that a personality clash is to do with personalities only. It does not cover any failings of your mentor in terms of their professional accountability and responsibility. These issues have been dealt with extensively in Chapter 3. If you feel that your mentor is not fulfilling their role, this should be raised with someone senior in the placement or a support lecturer from your university. A personality clash is separate from these types of issues and is simply a failure of two individuals to get along, rather than a failure in mentorship requirements.

A personality clash alone is not enough to justify a change of mentor. To change mentors just because you are not getting along resolves nothing, and only serves to avoid a situation that has the potential to be resolved. This is not to say that a personality clash should be trivialised, as your motivation to learn within a placement will almost certainly be compromised if you are not getting along with your mentor. However, putting this into some perspective, it is not reasonable to assume that you will be able to avoid personality clashes simply because they are difficult. What will you do if you do not particularly like the personality of your patients? Is it reasonable that you will be able to avoid patients you don't like, or who don't like you? The answer, of course, is a definite 'No'. This means that you will need to try to resolve personality clashes with mentors, as in doing so you will also be learning valuable skills of communication and negotiation.

The first thing to say is that it is possible to resolve personality clashes. Have a look again at Chapter 8 and the Johari window in Activity 8.1 on page 88. The second window represents what we may not know about ourselves, but others know about us. Without any doubt, there may be aspects of your character or personality that can annoy or irritate others. You will have no way of knowing what it is about your personality that a mentor may find irritating before you meet them, just as they will have no idea what you may dislike about them.

CASE STUDY 9.3

A mentor speaks about resolving a personality clash with a student:

A few years ago I was mentoring a student doing a theatre placement. We were always polite to each other and I didn't think there were any problems, but one day she asked to speak to me and I could see she was really upset. Then she tells me that it really upsets her when I ignore her in the morning. I explained that I'm not a morning person and I don't really like chatting in the morning, not until I've had a coffee anyway. I hadn't even realised I was ignoring her and felt really guilty when she pointed it out. We had a good laugh about it and the next day she even brought us both a latte. We had no more problems after that; we just needed to talk it through. Actually, I'm glad she pointed it out. I make a real effort now every morning not to come across so grumpy, which I'm sure everyone appreciates.

In some cases the personality clash you experience may be related to the fact that your mentor has a very different learning style from yours. Perhaps you are a reflector by nature and in your learning approach. If your mentor is more of an activist, this can lead to conflict and misunderstandings. Your mentor may misinterpret your preference for reflecting before acting as laziness or boredom. You, in turn, may misinterpret their desire for you to become more involved in activities as pushiness. Yet, whatever the reason, the only way you will be able to understand the origin of the personality clash is through communication. Remember, you don't have to become best friends with your mentor, you just need to find a way to work and learn together without conflict. If you fail to resolve these conflicts, your motivation for learning in practice will be compromised.

Learning with a disability

In 2007, the Nursing and Midwifery Admissions Service (NMAS) reported that over 1,200 students with known disabilities were accepted on to pre-registration nursing and/or midwifery courses in the UK (NMAS, 2007). As you can see in Table 9.1, these statistics make for some interesting reading.

Table 9.1: Applicants and acceptances by disability.

Disability	Number of applicants	Number of acceptances
No disability	21,865	11,520
Learning disability	592	323
Blind/partially sighted	37	20
Deaf/partial hearing	84	48
Wheelchair/mobility	16	11
Mental health	102	55
Unseen disability	196	104
Multiple disabilities	25	13
Other disability	180	97
Autistic disorder	1	0
Not known	624	572
Total	23,722	12,763

Source: NMAS (2007).

Given that some students may not be aware of their disability on entry to the programme, or choose not to disclose their disability, this number is almost certainly much higher. The point here is that, if you are undertaking the nursing course and do have a disability, you are certainly not unique. Many students just like you will be in the same position of needing to cope with the challenges of a disability while undertaking clinical placement. Obviously, the types of disabilities will be diverse and may include physical, mental or learning disabilities.

What do we mean by disability?

In 1995, the Disability and Discrimination Act (DDA) was introduced into legislation with the intention of protecting the rights of those with disabilities. According to this act, it an offence to discriminate against an individual because of their disability (DDA, 1995). Within this act a disability was classed as:

- a mental or physical impairment that has an adverse effect on the ability to carry out normal day-to-day activities;
- [and where] the adverse effect is substantial and long-term, meaning it has lasted for 12 months or is likely to last for 12 months more.

Since the original DDA 1995, there have been several amendments to the act that have relevance within nursing and particularly nursing and midwifery education. These include:

- 1995 Disability and Discrimination Act;
- 2001 Special Educational Needs and Disability Act;
- 2004 Amendment to Disability and Discrimination Act 1995;
- 2005 Disability and Discrimination Act.

The sum total of all these various acts of parliament means that a person with a disability should not be excluded from an educational opportunity as a result of that disability. In particular, the 2001 Special Educational Needs and Disability Act makes it unlawful for a disabled student to be excluded from a university course or programme because of their disability if they meet the entry requirements and professional/academic standards can be maintained.

In addition, the 2004 amendment to the DDA 1995 puts a duty on placement providers to make reasonable adjustments for disabled students, and to this end the NMC has been required to ensure that professional standards for entry to the professional register are objectively justifiable.

Finally, the DDA 2005 states that all publicly funded bodies (i.e. universities) are required to provide a disability scheme for the promotion and implementation of disability equality in their organisation.

What does this legislation mean for me?

The important thing to understand is that a student in the UK who has met entry criteria for a course of study is legally entitled to undertake each element of that study course without discrimination. In other words, your disability cannot be used as a reason to either include you, or to exclude you from commencing your nursing study. However, there is an important distinction that needs to be made here. An entitlement to undertake a study course is not, and should never be mistaken for, an entitlement for passing the course of study. Your disability is not a free ticket for passing. In other words, it is not discriminatory to fail a student with a disability on a course of study if they have not met the 'pass' criteria. However, the DDA 2005 does oblige a university or practice placement to make reasonable adjustments for a student with a disability, in order to ensure fairness and equality.

What are reasonable adjustments?

A reasonable adjustment is one that a university or practice placement might reasonably be expected to make in order to ensure that your disability is not preventing you from undertaking the study requirements of the course. You can expect that adjustments will be made to ensure that you are not discriminated against during your practice placement, although you should not expect to pass your placement objectives without demonstrating the necessary level of competence. For disabled students, this can mean that clinical practice can be a daunting and challenging experience. You may need to overcome a number of obstacles related to your disability in order to succeed. This may in turn affect your motivation.

Confidentiality and self-disclosure of your disability

There is no law that says that you must disclose your disability to anyone during the course of your nursing programme. This includes your mentor during your practice placement. Such information is classified as sensitive personal information and is covered by the Data Protection Act 1998. For this same reason, your university is not legally allowed to notify the placement area of your disability, nor do you have to disclose this information to the university. However, if you have chosen not to disclose your disability, the university is under no obligation to make reasonable adjustments that may ordinarily apply to your disability. Likewise, your mentor in practice and the placement provider are under no legal obligation to make reasonable adjustments if you do not make them aware of your disability. This means that the only way a mentor can know of your disability is if you tell them.

CASE STUDY 9.4

Rachel is a second-year student about to commence her clinical placement. She has dyslexia, and this was only discovered during her first year of training. So far, she has chosen not to disclose her disability for fear of being labelled. During school years Rachel was often ridiculed for being slow and she doesn't want the same treatment from her mentor. Much to Rachel's surprise, she discovers that her mentor also has dyslexia, and she realises that, in disclosing her disability, she is able to access help from her university. If Rachel had chosen not to inform her mentor of her disability, additional help and support would not have been available. Rachel has a great placement; the help she receives reduces her anxiety and allows her to maintain motivation.

The role of my mentor

If you do choose to disclose your disability, help will be made available to you. This is the law now, and there is legislation to protect your rights and prevent discrimination. Some of the help you receive in relation to your disability will be channelled via your mentor. It should be pointed out, however, that your mentor is not automatically required to know the exact nature of the reasonable adjustments that may be required for each student with a disability, or your special circumstances. In order to assist you in their role, the *Standards to Support Learning and Assessment in Practice* (NMC, 2008) require that your mentor must be provided with university support to ensure that they fulfil their professional and legal obligation in mentoring a student with a disability. However, once the reasonable adjustments are made clear, your mentor is required to facilitate these adjustments.

CHAPTER SUMMARY

Throughout all your placement experiences there will be times when you are faced with obstacles that have the potential to impact on your learning experience. Unless you can overcome these obstacles, your motivation to take full advantage of your supernumerary role and engage with all learning experiences will be compromised. You will need to develop both intrinsic and extrinsic motivational drivers that will sustain you through a wide variety of challenges, be it coping with the demands of shift work or juggling your home and family life around the structure of clinical placement. In addition, there will be personal issues that arise, personality clashes and/or coping with a disability. The good news is that, no matter what the challenges, there are practical solutions that you can develop to override the difficulties. By using these strategies you can maintain motivation to learn in, through and during practice placement.

KNOWLEDGE REVIEW

Having completed the chapter, how would you now rate your knowledge of the following topics?

	Good	Adequate	Poor
1. The various factors that affect motivation.			
2. The difference between intrinsic and extrinsic motivation.			
3. The common threats to motivation within clinical practice.			
4. The strategies you can use for getting motivated and staying motivated to learn in practice.			

Where you're not confident in your knowledge of a topic, what will you do next?

Further reading

Disability and Discrimination Act (DDA) (2005) Available online at **www.opsi.gov.uk/acts/acts2005/20050013.htm**.
The full act explains in detail the current legislation related to disability in the UK and implications for the public and private sector.

Useful websites

www.equalityhumanrights.com This is a useful website for current information about rights in different settings.
www.opsi.gov.uk/acts The Office of Public Sector Information website contains all UK Parliament Public General Acts from 1988 onwards, including all disability and discrimination acts.

andragogical a broad term that is used to describe learning strategies focused on how adults learn; it can also refer to the processes that are used to engage adult learners in the structure of the learning experience

experiential learning the process of making meaning and thereby learning through direct experiences

extrinsic motivation a desire to improve, or to achieve or attain a goal that is related to a specific reward

fitness for purpose an expectation by the NMC that, at the point of qualification, nurses must be able to relate to the changing needs of the health services and the communities that they serve, responding to current and future need in terms of provision of care, management of care, a health-for-all orientation and lifelong learning

high-road transfer the non-automatic examination of a situation with the aim of generating an alternative action when faced with an unfamiliar task

intrinsic motivation an internal desire to improve, or to achieve or attain a goal

knowledgeable doer a student who, after pre-registration education, should be able, on registration, to apply knowledge, understanding and skills when performing to the standards required in employment

low-road transfer skills that have been developed and can be used automatically with little conscious deliberation

Maslow's hierarchy of needs a predetermined group of motivating factors developed by Abraham Maslow, listed in order and levels of importance

mentor a registrant who has met the requirements of the NMC mentorship standard and is responsible and accountable for facilitating learning and assessing competence of students in a practice setting

motivation the reasons and/or principles behind why humans act, respond or perform in certain ways, including the drivers for making decisions

rostered service the final 20 per cent of practice placement time spent, prior to 1999, by pre-registration students; for the first 80 per cent, they had supernumerary status

self-direction an approach that relies heavily on students being responsible for their own learning; components can include distance programmes, blended learning, learning logs, learning contracts or problem-based packages

self-regulation an individual's ability to attain personalised academic goals through the use of proactive, self-directed internal and external strategies.

sign-off mentor an appropriately qualified nurse, midwife or health visitor who signs off students at the final assessment of practice, and confirms to the NMC that the required competencies for entry to the register have been achieved

supernumerary in relation to students, this means that they shall not, as part of their programme of preparation, be employed by any persons or body under a contract of service to provide nursing care; students are considered to be additional to the workforce requirements and staffing establishment figures

Allen, C (2002) Peers and partners: a stakeholder evaluation of preceptorship in mental health nursing. *Nurse Researcher*, 9(3): 68–84.

Andrews, M and Roberts, D (2003) Supporting student nurses learning in and through clinical practice: the role of the clinical guide. *Nurse Education Today*, 23: 474–81.

Aston, L and Molassiotis, A (2003) Supervising and supporting student nurses in clinical placements: the peer support intuitive. *Nurse Education Today*, 23: 202–10.

Atkins, S and Williams, A (1995) Registered nurses' experiences and mentoring undergraduate nursing students. *Journal of Advanced Nursing*, 21: 1006–15.

Baard, P and Neville, S (1996) The intrinsically motivated nurse: help and hindrance from evaluation feedback sessions. *Journal of Nursing Administration*, 26(7/8): 19–26.

Beck, C (1993) Nursing students' initial clinical experience: a phenomenological study. *International Journal of Nursing Studies*, 30(6): 489–97.

Begley, C and Brady, A (2002) Irish diploma in nursing students' first clinical allocation: the views of nurse managers. *Journal of Nursing Management*, 10: 339–47.

Begley, C and White, P (2003) Irish nursing students' changing self-esteem and fear of negative evaluation during their preregistration programme. *Journal of Advanced Nursing*, 42(4): 390–401.

Benabou, R and Tirole, J (2003) Intrinsic and extrinsic motivation. *Review of Economic Studies*, 70: 489–520.

Boud, D, Cohen, R and Walker, D (1993) *Using Experience for Learning.* Buckingham: The Society for Research into Higher Education and Open University Press.

Cahill, H (1996) A qualitative analysis of student nurses' experiences of mentorship. *Journal of Advanced Nursing*, 24: 791–9.

Cantor, J (1995) *Experiential Learning in Higher Education.* Washington, DC: The George Washington University.

Carroll, M, Curtis, L, Higgins, A, Nicholl, H, Redmond, R and Timmins, F (2001) Is there a place for reflective practice in the nursing curriculum? *Nurse Education in Practice*, 2: 13–20.

Chambers, M (1998) Some issues in the assessment of clinical practice: a review of the literature. *Journal of Clinical Nursing*, 7(3): 201–8.

Clynes, M (2008) Providing feedback on clinical performance to student nurses in children's nursing: challenges facing preceptors. *Journal of Children's and Young People's Nursing*, 2(1): 29–35.

Clynes, M and Raftery, S (2008) Feedback: an essential element of student learning in clinical practice. *Nurse Education in Practice*, 8(6): 405–11.

Corder, N (2008) *Learning to Teach Adults: An Introduction*, 2nd edition. London: Routledge.

Crawford, D (2004) The role of aging in adult learning: implications for instructors in higher education. *New Horizons for Learning.* Available online at www.new horizons.org/lifelong/higher_ed/crawford.htm (accessed 23 December 2008).

Davies, B, Neary, M and Phillips, R (1994) *The Practitioner-Teacher.* Cardiff: School of Education, University of Wales.

Dawson, C (2006) *The Mature Student's Study Guide*. Oxford: How To Books.

Delahaye, B and Ehrich, L (2008) Complex learning preferences and strategies of older adults. *Educational Gerontology*, 34(8): 649–62.

Dennison, B and Kirk, R (1990) *Do, Review, Learn, Apply: A simple guide to experiential learning*. Oxford: Blackwell Education.

Dewey, J (1933*) How We Think: A restatement of the relation of reflective thinking to the educative process.* New York: Heath and Co.

Disability and Discrimination Act (DDA) (1995) Available online at www.opsi.gov.uk/acts/acts1995/1995050.htm (accessed 26 February 2009).

Disability and Discrimination Act (DDA)(1995) (Amendment 2004) Available online at www.opsi.gov.uk.si/si2003/draft/20035776.htm (accessed 13 February 2009).

Disability and Discrimination Act (DDA) (2005) Available online at www.opsi.gov.uk/acts/acts2005/20050013.htm (accessed 26 February 2009).

Dohrenwend, A (2002) Serving up the feedback sandwich. *Family Practice Management*, 9(10): 43–9.

Duley, J (1980) *Learning Outcomes: The measurement and evaluation of experiential learning*. Washington, DC: National Society for Internships and Experiential Education.

Dunn, R and Dunn, K (1999) *The Complete Guide to the Learning Styles Inservice System.* Boston, MA: Allyn and Bacon.

Eaton, L (1995) A clinical evaluation tool that gives students feedback. *Nurse Educator*, 20(3): 9–10.

Elcock, K (2006) Wake up and learn. *Nursing Standard*, 20(49): 61.

Elcock, K (2007) Where there's smoke. *Nursing Standard*, 21(44): 61.

Elcock, K, Curtis, P and Sharples, K (2007) Supernumerary status: an unrealised ideal. *Nurse Education in Practice*, 7: 4–10.

Eraut, M (2006) Editorial. *Learning in Health and Social Care*, 5(3): 111–18.

Fitzpatrick, J, While, A and Roberts, J (1996) Key influences on the professional socialisation and practice of students undertaking different pre-registration nurse education programmes in the United Kingdom. *International Journal of Nursing Studies*, 33(5): 506–18.

Flanagan, J, Baldwin, S and Clarke, D (2000) Work-based learning as a means of developing and assessing nursing competence. *Journal of Clinical Nursing*, 9: 360–8.

Fleming, J and Courtney, B (1984) The dimensionality of self-esteem II. Hierarchical facet model for revised measurement scales. *Journal of Personality and Social Psychology*, 46: 404–21.

Ghaye, T and Lillyman, S (eds) (2000) *Effective Clinical Supervision: The role of Reflection.* Salisbury: Quay Books.

Ghaye, T and Lillyman, S (2008) *The Reflective Mentor.* London: Quay Books.

Ghaye, T, Cuthbert, S, Danai, K and Dennis, D (1996) *An Introduction to Learning through Critical Reflective Practice: Self-supported learning experiences for healthcare professionals.* Newcastle upon Tyne: Pentaxion Press.

Glover, P (2000) 'Feedback. I listened, reflected and utilized': third year nursing students' perceptions and use of feedback in the clinical setting. *International Journal of Nursing Practice*, 6: 247–52.

Gray, M and Smith, L (1999) The professional socialization of diploma of higher education in nursing students (Project 2000): a longitudinal qualitative study. *Journal of Advanced Nursing*, 29(3): 639–47.

Gray, M and Smith, L (2000) The qualities of an effective mentor from the student nurse's perspective: findings from a longitudinal study. *Journal of Advanced Nursing*, 32(6): 1542–9.

Haidar, E (2007) Coaching and mentoring nursing students. *Nursing Management*, 14(8): 32–5.

Harvey, T and Vaughan, J (1990) Student nurses' attitudes towards different teaching/learning methods. *Nurse Education Today*, 10: 181–5.

Hayes, A (2006) *Teaching Adults.* London: Continuum.

Honey, P and Mumford, A (1989) *The Manual of Learning Opportunities.* Maidenhead: Peter Honey Publications.

Honey, P and Mumford, A (1992) *The Manual of Learning Styles*. Maidenhead: Peter Honey Publications. Peter Honey Publications would like us to note that this publication is now out of print but has been replaced by: Honey, P and Mumford, A (2006) *The Learning Styles Questionnaire, 80-item version*. Maidenhead: Peter Honey Publications. Page references in this book relate to the 1992 edition.

Honey, P and Mumford, A (1995) *Using Your Learning Style*. Maidenhead: Peter Honey Publications.

Howard, S (1993) Accreditation of prior learning: andragogy in action or a 'cut price' approach to education? *Journal of Advanced Nursing*, 18: 1817–24.

Jarvis, P (1992) Reflective practice and nursing. *Nurse Education Today*, 12(3): 174–81.

Johnson, D and Preston, B (2001) *An Overview of Issues in Nursing Education.* Department of Education, Science and Training, Australia. Available online at www.pandora.nla.gov.au/pan/23224/20020121-0000/www.detya.gov.au/highered/eippubs/eip01_12/fullreport.htm (accessed 23 December 2008).

Kelly, C (2007) Students' perceptions of effective clinical teaching revisited. *Nurse Education Today*, 27: 885–92.

Kelly, D, Sharples, K and Elcock, K (2007) Take direct action. *Nursing Standard*, 21(22): 61.

Kilbourne, B (1990) *Constructive Feedback: Learning the art.* Toronto, Ontario: Ontario Institute for Studies in Education.

Kilminster, S, Cottrell, D, Grant, J and Jolly, B (2007) AMEE guide No 27: Effective educational and clinical supervision. *Medical Teacher*, 29: 2–19.

Knowles, M (1984) *Andragogy in Action.* San Francisco, CA: Jossey-Bass.

Knowles, M (1989) *The Making of an Adult Educator.* San Francisco, CA: Jossey-Bass.

Knowles, M (1990) *The Adult Learner: A neglected species*, 4th edition. Houston, TX: Gulf.

Knowles, M, Holton, E and Swanson, R (1998) *The Adult Learner*, 5th edition. Houston, TX: Gulf.

Knowles, M, Holton, E and Swanson, R (2005) *The Adult Learner*, 6th edition. London: Elsevier.

Kolb, D (1984) *Experiential Learning: Experience as the source of learning and development.* Mahwah, NJ: Prentice Hall.

Li, S, Chen, P and Tsai, S (2008) A comparison of the learning styles among different nursing programmes in Taiwan: implications for nursing education. *Nurse Education Today*, 28: 70–6.

Lofmark, A and Wikblad, K (2001) Facilitating and obstructing factors for development of learning in clinical practice: a student perspective. *Journal of Advanced Nursing*, 34(1): 43–50.

London, M (1995) Giving feedback: Source-centered antecedents and consequences of constructive and destructive feedback. *Human Resource Management Review*, 5(3): 159–88.

MacLeod, M (1995) What does it mean to be well taught? A hermeneutic course evaluation. *Journal of Nursing Education*, 34(5): 197–203.

Maitland, I (1995) *Motivating People*. Guernsey, CI: The Guernsey Press.

Maslow, A (1943) A theory of human motivation. *Psychological Review*, 50: 370–96.

Maslow, A (1987) *Motivation and Personality*, 3rd edition. New York: Harper and Row.

McMillan, M and Dwyer, J (1990) Facilitating a match between teaching and learning styles. *Nurse Education Today*, 10: 186–92.

Mezirow, J (1983) A critical theory of adult learning and education, in Tight, M (ed) *Education for Adults: Educational opportunities for adults*. Beckenham: Croom Helm in association with the Open University.

Mullen, P (2007) Use of self-regulating learning strategies by students in the second and third trimesters of an accelerated second-degree baccalaureate nursing programme. *Journal of Nursing Education*, 46(9): 406–11.

Murphy, K and Atkins, S (1994) Reflection with a practice-led curriculum, in Palmer, A, Burns, S and Bulman, C (eds) *Reflective Practice in Nursing: The growth of the professional practitioner*. Oxford: Blackwell Scientific.

Myers, I (1995) *Gifts Differing*. Palo Alto, CA: Consulting Psychologists Press.

Myers, I, McCaulley, M, Quenk, N and Hammer, A (1998) *MBTI Manual: A guide to the development and use of the Myers-Briggs Type Indicator*, 3rd edition. Palo Alto, CA: Consulting Psychologists Press.

Nursing and Midwifery Admissions Service (NMAS) (2007) *Statistical Report 2007*. Available online at www.nmas.ac.uk (accessed 28 October 2008).

Nursing and Midwifery Council (NMC) (2004) *Standards of Proficiency for Pre-registration Nursing Education*. London: NMC.

Nursing and Midwifery Council (NMC) (2007) *Essential Skills Clusters for Pre-registration Nursing Programmes*. London: NMC.

Nursing and Midwifery Council (NMC) (2008) *Standards to Support Learning and Assessment in Practice: NMC standards for mentors, practice teachers and teachers*. London: NMC.

Pattison, D, Parsons, D and Weatherhead, C (2000) Connecting reflective practice with clinical supervision. In Ghaye, T and Lilliman, S (eds) *Effective Clinical Supervision: The role of reflection*. London: Quay Books.

Pearce, C (2004) Giving and receiving feedback. *Nursing Times*, 100(50): 46–7.

Pugh, B (1992) Feedback in clinical teaching. *Nurse Educator*, 17(1): 5–7.

Rogers, C (1983) *Freedom to Learn for the 80's*. London: Merrill Publishing Company.

Rogers, J (2007) *Adults Learning*. Maidenhead: Open University Press.

Royal College of Nursing (RCN) (2005) *Guidance for Mentors of Student Nurses and Midwives: An RCN toolkit*. London: RCN.

Royal College of Nursing (RCN) (2007) *Guidance for Mentors of Student Nurses and Midwives: An RCN toolkit*. London: RCN.

Russell, T (1994) *Effective Feedback Skills*. London: Kogan.

Salomon, G and Perkins, D (1989) Rocky roads to transfer: rethinking mechanisms of a neglected phenomenon. *Educational Psychologist*, 24: 113–42.

Schon, D (1983) *The Reflective Practitioner*. New York: Basic Books.

Sharples, K (2006) Shifting priorities. *Nursing Standard*, 21(8): 61.

Sharples, K (2007a) Are you just the job? *Nursing Standard*, 21(40): 61.

Sharples, K (2007b) Sign for success. *Nursing Standard*, 21(51): 64.

Sharples, K (2007c) Supporting nursing students. *Nursing Standard*, 21(50): 64.

Sharples, K and Kelly, D (2006) A hard day's night. *Nursing Standard*, 21(4): 61.

Sharples, K, Kelly, D and Elcock, K (2007) Supporting mentors in practice. *Nursing Standard*, 21(39): 44–7.

Smedley, A (2007) The self-directed learning readiness of first year Bachelor of Nursing students. *Journal of Research in Nursing*, 12(4): 373–85.

Special Educational Needs and Disability Act (2001) Available online at www.opsi.gov.uk/acts/acts2001/20010010.htm (accessed 16 January 2009).

Spouse, J (2003) *Professional Learning in Nursing*. Oxford: Blackwell Science.

Steves, A (2005) Improving the clinical instruction of student technologists. *Journal of Nuclear Medicine Technology*, 33(4): 205–9.

Stryjewski, G and Slonim, A (2002) Who says you're too tired? *Critical Care Medicine*, 30(10): 2396–7.

Sung, K (2006) Literature review on self-regulated learning. *Singapore Nursing Journal*, 33(2): 38–45.

Timmins, F (2008) *Making Sense of Portfolios: A guide for nursing students*. Maidenhead: Open University Press.

UK Central Council for Nursing Midwifery and Health Visiting (UKCC) (1986) *Project 2000: A new preparation for practice*. London: UKCC.

UK Central Council for Nursing Midwifery and Health Visiting (UKCC) (1999) *Fitness for Practice: The UKCC Commission for Nursing and Midwifery Education*. London: UKCC.

Vernon, M (1969) *Human Motivation*. Cambridge: Cambridge University Press.

Watson, R, Stimpson, A, Topping, A and Porock, D (2002) Clinical competence assessment in nursing: a systematic review of the literature. *Journal of Advanced Nursing*, 39(5): 421–31.

Wiggins, G (1998) *Educative Assessment: Designing assessment to inform and improve student performance*. San Francisco, CA: Jossey-Bass.

Wilkinson, C, Peters, L, Mitchell, K, Irwin, T, McCorrie, K and Macleod, M (1998) 'Being there': learning through active participation. *Nurse Education Today*, 18: 226–30.

Windsor, A (1987) Nursing students' perceptions of clinical experience. *Journal of Nursing Education*, 26(4): 150–4.

Withnall, A, McGivney, V and Soulsby, J (2004) *Older People Learning: Myths and realities*. Leicester: NIACE.

Yong, V (1996) 'Doing clinical': The lived experience of nursing students. *Contemporary Nurse*, 5: 73–9.

Young, P (2000) 'I might as well give up': self-esteem and mature students' feelings about feedback on assignments. *Journal of Further and Higher Education*, 24(3): 409–18.

Zimmerman, B (1995) Self-regulation involves more than meta-cognition: a social cognitive perspective. *Educational Psychologist*, 30: 217–22.

Index

A
absences 58
abstract conceptualisation 80–1, 93
accountability, mentors 30, 32–3
active experimentation 81–2, 93
'activist' learning style 41, 44, 46, 82
adult learners 17–18, 38, 44
    andragogy 19–20, 114
    characteristics 18
    core principles 20–1
    learning in practice 23–4
    positive/negative experiences 21–2
    see also learning styles
affective skills 32
age, and learning 17–18, 44
andragogy 19–20, 114
anxiety, clinical placement 49–52
assessment in practice 31–2, 32–3
    see also feedback
audit trail, assessment 96

B
Boud, David 74

C
clinical placement 49
    and disability 109–12
    feelings prior to 49–51
    planning for learning 52–6
    practice versus theory 63–4
    preparation for 51–2, 56–60
    see also feedback; learning
    activities/experiences; mentors
clusters, essential skills *see*
    Essential Skills Clusters for
    Pre-registration Nursing
    Programmes
cognitive skills 32
Commission for Education 8
competence
    aspects of 31–2, 63
    assessment of 32–3
    and learning styles 47

levels of 12, 32
    see also feedback
conceptualisation, abstract 80–1, 93
concrete experience 77–8, 93
confidentiality, and disability 111–12
constructive feedback 92
continuing professional development
    (CPD) 2, 3, 7, 12
critical reflection 80
curriculum design 13–15
    andragogy 19–20, 114

D
Data Protection Act 112
DDA *see* Disability and
    Discrimination Act
Dennison, Bill 88
descriptive reflection 79
disability, and learning 109–12
Disability and Discrimination Act
    (DDA) 110–11
discrimination, disability 111
documentation, feedback 95–6

E
Eraut, Michael 86
Essential Skills Clusters for
    Pre-registration Nursing
    Programmes 1, 3, 10, 12–13,
    32, 75
experiential learning cycle 76–7, 114
    abstract conceptualisation 80–1, 93
    active experimentation 81–2, 93
    concrete experience 77–8, 93
    and feedback 93–4
    and learning styles 82
    reflective observation 78–80, 93
experimentation, active 81–2, 93
extrinsic motivation 103, 104–5, 114

F
facilitation of learning 30–1
family life, and shift work 57, 107